With *Eat Well, Move Well, Live Well*, readers benefit from a method as simple as it is powerful. By adopting a series of manageable habits and focusing on building awareness, readers of this book will be set up to finally achieve sustainable success. In a sea of fitness confusion, this an oasis of sanity.

—Mark Fisher, Mark Fisher Fitness

With their latest book, *Eat Well Move Well Live Well*, Roland and Galina Denzel offer a down-to-earth roadmap for a lifestyle over-haul. They enthusiastically touch on a little of everything, high-lighting the important fact that "lifestyle" isn't just what we eat or how long we exercise…there's so much more.

—Angelo Coppola, creator of the *Latest in Paleo* podcast, the *Humans Are Not Broken* blog, and *The Plant Paleo Diet*

Eat Well, Move Well, Live Well is a light-hearted and personal journey through many important aspects of health and well-being. Roland and Galina Denzel pull together research, personal experience, and a hefty dose of common sense to help us live better in the modern world.

—Stephan Guyenet, PhD

An informative and helpful book that is also fun. The Denzels offer practical guidance on how to take advantage of cutting-edge health information, all while making it easy to see big-picture ways to improve your life.

—Dan Pardi, MS, PhD(c), CEO, humanOS.me.
Research with Zeitzer Lab at Stanford University,
and Dept. of Neurology and Endocrinology
at Leiden University, Netherlands.

Well-written, relatable, and most importantly full of tips for doing stuff right away, this book covers pretty much everything you need to know to live, eat, play, and just *be* better. Don't be fooled by the friendly tone; this book is experience- and evidence-based, full of solid advice you can use immediately.

—Krista Scott-Dixon, PhD

Roland and Galina have put together an amazingly useful book here, since the information is both accurate and actionable, which is a rare one-two punch. It walks you through a great background on each area with just enough information to make it relevant without too much fluff, and just enough action to make it doable. I highly recommend you pick up this book and put it into practice. I know you will be better for it.

—Mike T. Nelson, CSCS, PhD

Roland and Galina Denzel have nailed it with this book. They've taken the complex and seemingly insurmountable task of "getting healthy," and broken it down into easy-to-understand – but more importantly, easy-to-implement – steps that allow the average person to start moving toward better health and a better life instantly. Roland and Galina's genuine passion for helping others shines through. This book is gold. If you want to start eating, moving, and living better, but have felt overwhelmed, let Roland and Galina show you the way.

- Molly Galbraith, owner, Girls Gone Strong

EAT WELL

MOVE WELL

LIVE WELL

52 WAYS TO FEEL BETTER IN A WEEK

ROLAND DENZEL & GALINA DENZEL

FOREWORD BY DR. SPENCER NADOLSKY

PROPRIOMETRICS
PRESS

Printed in the United States of America.
First Printing, 2016
ISBN-13: 978-1-943370-02-3
Library of Congress Control Number: 2016940675
Propriometrics Press: propriometricspress.com
Cover and Interior Design: Zsofi Koller, zsofikoller.com
Photography: J. Jurgensen Photography and Adobe Stock
Illustrator: Elmira Nam
Author Photo Photographer: Shannon Leith

Publisher's Cataloging-In-Publication Data
(Prepared by The Donohue Group, Inc.)

Names: Denzel, Roland. | Denzel, Galina.
Title: Eat well, move well, live well : 52 ways to feel better in a week /
Roland Denzel & Galina Denzel.
Description: [Sequim, Washington] : Propriometrics Press, [2016] |
Includes bibliographical references and index.
Identifiers: LCCN 2016940675 | ISBN 978-1-943370-02-3 |
   ISBN 978-1-943370-06-1 (ebook)
Subjects: LCSH: Health. | Well-being. | Human mechanics.
Classification: LCC RA776.95 .D46 2016 (print) | LCC RA776.95 (ebook)
| DDC 613--dc23

The information in this book should not be used for diagnosis or treatment,
or as a substitute for professional medical care. Please consult with your
health-care provider prior to attempting any treatment on yourself or
another individual.

CONTENTS

FOREWORD

I have been passionate about health and wellness for more than seventeen years, and as a doctor, I'm proud to prescribe lifestyle as medicine.

As a physician specializing in obesity, my goal is to improve my patients' lifestyles so that they are successful in losing weight and keeping it off. And as the "Doc Who Lifts," I like to demonstrate that I practice what I preach. I want people to be empowered to make change, live healthily, and feel good in their bodies and lives, but there are so many obstacles to good health today.

We live in a culture obsessed with appearance and youth, not health. We're disconnected from our food. We don't cook it much ourselves anymore, much less grow it. Our communities are being replaced by online friendships, and our movement habits are more about clicking and scrolling than walking and playing. Most of us sit in front of a screen day and night. I'll bet most people see more sunsets and friends on social media than they do in real life.

Most of us know change needs to happen. Many want to change, but once a habit is ingrained – once you've become sedentary, a television or screen junky, or a regular junk food eater – changing habits is hard, especially when you don't know where to start.

Habits, in fact, are why this book, *Eat Well, Move Well, Live Well*, is so important. It's not a gimmick or a get-healthy-quick scheme. This is a guide to making small but powerful changes, ones modest enough that they aren't overwhelming or too difficult, but meaningful enough to quietly overhaul even the least healthy lifestyle.

Practically everyone – whether they're eating fast food three times a day or growing their own veggies and cooking from scratch – has gaps in their health that could stand improvement. Whether it's by eating mindfully, cooking new dishes, moving or exercising more, or just getting better sleep, Roland and Galina are ready to help you become the healthiest possible version of yourself.

Several years ago, the three of us met and became friends at The Fitness Summit in Kansas City. We found that we have many goals and ideas in common, and we are always striving to learn how to help our clients. We have different specialties, but in the end, it's the long-term health of our clients and patients that matters to each of us.

I'm so glad to have this empowering, enlightening book available to give to my patients.

—Dr. Spencer Nadolsky

PREFACE

Writing this book has transformed us. People think that health coaches are the living incarnation of all that we teach – we go to bed early, get up with the sunrise, and never lose our temper. We drink bone broth instead of coffee, bathe in Epsom salts, hold hands and forgive each other easily all while walking into a warm California sunset.

This utopian idea forgets one thing – we are human. We are human animals who live in the same environment as our clients; we have jobs, smartphones, deadlines, extended families, and children. We go to school, go to the doctor, and go crazy the same way our clients do. We navigate the same supermarkets, traffic jams, and holiday potlucks. Our bellies bloat, we get gassy, we have sucky days, tend to isolate, and get addicted to technology and work.

It's true that being immersed in health information through our work keeps us more conscious and makes it easier to stay healthy, but just like our clients, we allow certain habits to develop and then notice, sometimes a bit late, that our minds, bodies, and relationships have started to suffer.

Writing this book, one chapter at a time, has allowed us to integrate the health habits that we teach our clients and has invited more positive growth in our minds, bodies, and relationships than we ever expected. When we started writing it we wanted to transform you – in the process, we got transformed. We invite you to read this book, whether from cover to cover, or starting at a chapter on a favorite subject, and allow it to work its magic.

We invite you to be curious about how one small step, such as learning how to make bone broth, or brushing your teeth in a new way, can bring profound change in your understanding of self-care and your ability to be physically empowered in an environment that actively robs you of your birthright to live well in your body, within a supporting community, and in connection with nature.

For some of you this book will be a journey that takes a few months or years; for others it will be a helpful troubleshooter that occupies your coffee table or nightstand. You can take it further – our website offers you several ways to engage, from supplementary videos and articles, to joining with others as passionate about health and wellness as you are. Join a group, start a challenge, and connect with a community of people who are adopting the same health habits as you are, or even working with us personally. You can engage as little or as much as you like, and you have our support in any path that you take on your journey. Let's go.

Roland & Galina

HOW TO USE THIS BOOK

This book is yours, and there is no right or wrong way to use it. You will find your way, and your way is always changing, because you are always changing.

That being said, we've identified three basic ways to start interacting with this book, choosing the paths on your journey to being well. Whichever way you choose, make sure that you start a paper or electronic journal where you can write down your thoughts and plans as they relate to the tasks in each chapter.

1. Read the book from start to finish

This is great for those of you who love to see the big picture. As you read each chapter, enjoy the content and note which chapters you would like to come back to and take action on. Some chapters may speak to you strongly, such as how to make great bone broth or brush your teeth better, and others, such as enjoying coffee, may not be your favorite cup at all. Reading through the whole book will give you an idea of the paths you want for your journey and will keep the map under your control.

2. Read one chapter at a time and "choose your own adventure"

Remember those books that took you on a wild ride way before the days of computer games? You would finish a chapter and take the hero to page 213 to find new exciting adventures waiting there. The end of each chapter in this book has two suggestions for chapters to go to afterward. This way you weave your way through the book keeping pace with a map designed by us. This is a great option for the thrill seekers among you.

If you've chosen to follow this style of reading, you'll notice that we handpicked the first four lessons for you. These four have been so important to our clients that we decided to recommend them as a great way to start before moving on to other lessons. These first four recommended lessons are:

Chapter 1: The Sunday Food Ritual (p.6)
Chapter 15: Tame Your Sugar Monster (p.110)
Chapter 45: Walk More Today (p.345)
Chapter 38: Your Dynamic Office (p.294)

3. Health troubleshooter

Look through the table of contents to determine those chapters you want to work on first. Unlike taking the fully guided approach and doing the whole book according to someone else's plan, you can choose to use the chapters that help you troubleshoot specific areas of your life, such as meditation, mindful eating, or planning your next vacation. Keep reading ahead – there's always more to find out about yourself.

Of course, there's always the "deck of cards" approach that we talked about earlier, for those who want to leave a little bit up to chance!

Make each chapter yours

Your paper or electronic journal can help you navigate the lessons and record your transformation. You can use a fancy, leather-bound journal, a composition book, a notepad app on your phone, or download the journal that we provide on our resources page. As you go through each chapter, open your journal and answer some questions, such as:

- What in this chapter speaks to you?
- How would you like to use this information for yourself now or later?
- What are some ways you have tried to incorporate this type of lesson before, and how were you successful or not?
- How will the information in this specific chapter benefit you and how will it benefit those around you?
- Do you commit to a time you want to practice this habit, such as several times a week or daily for a couple of months? Establish a date when you can come back to this journal entry and record your results.

We worked hard to keep each chapter short and sweet, but there was always more we wanted to share, so we've created a page on our website just for that. Head over to eatmovelive52.com for additional resources for each chapter, from recipes and tips, to articles and books, videos for the exercises, interviews with our experts, and even ways to find professionals in your area.

Join the community

Galina teaches a weekly walking group called "Never Walk Alone."

We believe that incremental changes are the way to grow, and small steps when done holding hands with others on the same path will stick the longest.

Head over to eatmovelive52.com to find others who are reading the book and working through habits of self-care and well-being. The journey with others will allow you to ask questions, get feedback on how you are doing, and interact with the coaches – we will be there to encourage you and support you in your transition, celebrate your success, and lift you up when you are down!

Grab your journal, or open a new page in your note-taking program, and let's go.

COOKING

1 The Sunday Food Ritual by Roland

*Save time, money, and calories by dedicating one day
per week to this week's meals*

Eating out can be expensive, but people do it anyway. Surveys show averages of up to 50% of some family food budgets are spent eating out. In a recent survey by Ally Bank, even the people who could afford it least often spent an average of 40% of their monthly food budget eating away from home.

These are just the averages, meaning that for every home chef who only eats out on special occasions, there's that guy who eats every meal out of the house, and for every family who eats a home-cooked meal each night, there's a family who hits the drive-through instead.

We're talking big differences, too. A meal purchased at a restaurant will often cost twice what it would when made at home, where you know what's going into it.

Yes, we know, but...

The costs of eating out quickly add up to a lot of wasted money, to plenty of empty calories, and to poor health and nutrition.

When asked why they choose to continue to eat out for so many of their meals, our readers, clients, and friends tell us that they simply don't know what to cook, or don't have the time to cook it; instead they rely on fast food on the way home, or pack up the family for an even more expensive trip to a sit-down restaurant.

We all want more time with family or friends, more money in our wallets at the end of the month, better health, and smaller waistlines, all while eating delicious foods. You can have all that and more, all by doing some simple planning, and shifting some of your cooking time from your busy weekdays to a slower Sunday afternoon.

I know, Sunday is supposed to be a day of rest, so the idea of packing even more into an already busy day is the last thing you want to hear, but with two parents working, busy kids' soccer schedules, errands to run, lawns to mow, and houses to clean, the rest of our week is already stuffed to the gills!

One of the most powerful things you can do to improve your family's bottom line is to consolidate some of your *daily* cooking time into a Sunday ritual, giving yourself back time on your weeknights. This ends up saving you money, and giving you better control of your family's health and nutrition. (Of course, if Saturday works better, or Wednesday night, do the ritual then.)

We'll start off easy. This week you're going to make a base meal from an inexpensive pork roast. You will not only get to eat it on Sunday night, but it will be the main ingredient for some delicious dinners later in the week. You might even have leftovers, which is a real bonus for those of us who pack lunches for the office!

Don't like pork? Make the same dish using chicken – thighs and breasts.

Three-in-One Slow Cooker Pork Recipe

Makes three dinners for four people
Day One – Slow Cooker Pork Roast and Veggies
Day Two – Pozole (Mexican Pork Stew)
Day Three – Carnitas Tacos or Carnitas Taco Salad

Day One – Slow Cooker Pork Roast and Veggies

I highly recommend a slow cooker, but you don't need to use a slow cooker to make any of these meals. They can really make life easier, but don't wait until you find the perfect model to start your Sunday ritual.

Slow cookers allow you to set the food to cook and then go about your day without stirring, prodding, and checking. If you don't have a slow cooker, any large, covered pot will work; you'll just have to stick around to monitor your progress.

You will need a pretty large slow cooker for this, but today's slow cookers are inexpensive. I recently purchased an 8-quart slow cooker at Target for about $35, but I've seen good ones as low as $20. I generally recommend that you get a 6- or 8-quart slow cooker, so you can make enough food for several meals at once.

Of the three, this is the only meal that you have to start well ahead of time. Cooking in a slow cooker is hands-off after you start it, but it does take time to prepare. Meals two and three will be much faster, after the slow work is done.

Serves 4

INGREDIENTS

- 4–5 pound pork roast (blade, butt, shoulder, etc.) or substitute chicken thighs and breasts
- 1 ½ pounds fingerling potatoes (fingerling or tiny red or white potatoes hold together better when slow cooking)
- 1 medium onion, cut into wedges
- 1 pound carrots, cut into large pieces
- 4 garlic cloves, minced or pressed
- 4 bay leaves

- 2 tbsp ground cumin
- 2 tbsp ground coriander
- 2 tbsp paprika
- 1 tbsp salt
- water

DIRECTIONS

1. Place the meat in the slow cooker, and nestle the vegetables around the sides. Sprinkle the herbs and spices over the top. Add enough water to cover the vegetables and meat.

2. Cook on high for six to seven hours or nine to ten hours on low. Times will vary based on the size of your roast and the size and model of your slow cooker.

3. Remove the meat to a platter or large bowl to rest for a few minutes before cutting it up. The roast, when done, will likely be tender enough to fall apart, so if having it whole is important to you, be careful lifting and transferring it.

4. Using a slotted spoon, transfer the vegetables to tonight's dinner plates. If desired, leave some or all of the onions in the broth for the pozole that you'll be making later in the week.

5. Remember that this is enough meat for three meals, so divide the meat into three portions.

6. Refrigerate one portion in a container to save for carnitas tacos.

7. Refrigerate a second portion and all of your broth to save for the pozole. The remaining third is for tonight, so cut that up and transfer to tonight's dinner plates.

Day Two – Pozole (Mexican Pork Stew)

Pozole is a brothy soup or stew, traditionally made with dried hominy in a huge caldron. You probably don't have a caldron, and dried hominy is almost impossible to find in this country, so just use a soup pot and canned hominy, which is available in most supermarkets in the canned vegetable section or the Hispanic foods section. If you can't find hominy, you can still make a delicious version of this soup with fresh or frozen yellow corn.

Serves 4

INGREDIENTS

- Reserved pork (or chicken) and broth
- 8 medium yellow summer squash and/or zucchini (mix and match), cut into circles
- 4 medium carrots, cut into thin circles
- 2 small cans hominy, drained or a 16-oz bag of frozen corn
- Salt to taste
- 1 tbsp dried oregano (Mexican oregano preferred, but not required)
- Green salsa (optional)
- Hot sauce (optional)

DIRECTIONS

1. Heat the broth and vegetables in a pot. If using canned hominy, add it now. If using corn, add it at the end so it doesn't overcook and lose its sweetness.

2. Add additional water, if necessary, to make sure you have enough broth to go around. I prefer it closer to soup than stew, but there's no right or wrong here. Bring the pot to a simmer and let the vegetables cook for about 15 minutes.

3. While the soup is simmering, cut or shred the pork into bite-size pieces.
4. When the vegetables are getting tender, stir in the meat. If using frozen corn, add it now. Bring it back to a simmer and let it cook for another 5–10 minutes until the corn and meat are heated through.
5. Salt to taste.
6. Just before serving, rub the oregano between your palms over the pot of soup, then ladle the soup into bowls.
7. Serve with green salsa and hot sauce on the side.

Day Three – Carnitas Tacos and Chopped Salad

Carnitas is slowly braised pork that is later pan fried and shredded. Carnitas makes great tacos, but if you don't want the carbs or calories of the tortillas, a bag of mixed greens turns carnitas tacos into a taco salad pretty easily!

Serves 4

INGREDIENTS

- 3–4 ripe tomatoes, chopped or 1 pint cherry tomatoes, chopped
- 1 yellow, orange, or red bell pepper, seeded and chopped
- 1 cucumber, peeled and chopped or 3–4 Persian cucumbers, chopped
- 1 tbsp olive oil
- Salt to taste
- 2 ripe avocados
- Reserved pork (or chicken)

- 1 tbsp fat (lard, bacon fat, butter, ghee) or oil (olive, coconut, or palm oil)
- 2–4 tortillas per person
- Red or green jarred salsa
- Sour cream (optional)
- Shredded cheddar or jack cheese (optional)
- 1 bag mixed greens (optional)

DIRECTIONS

1. Make the chopped salad by stirring the tomatoes, peppers, and cucumber together. Stir in the olive oil, salt to taste, and set aside.

2. Mash the avocados and set them aside.

3. Shred or cut the pork into bite size pieces. Heat the fat or oil over medium high heat, and add the pork, stirring and flipping periodically to heat it through and produce a few crispy bits, if desired. Remove from heat, set aside, and start cooking the tortillas.

4. I learned a special method for heating corn tortillas when I was in Mexico, and although it's a little more work, they hold together a lot better than steamed ones. If you're short for time, you can simply wrap them in a damp towel and steam them, but I hope you'll try my method at least once:

   Get a bowl that's big enough for dipping a tortilla, fill it with water, and set it near the stove. Heat a large non-stick skillet over medium-high to high heat. When the skillet is very hot, dip the tortilla in the water, and put it on the skillet. Let it sit and sizzle until it can be *easily* lifted with a spatula (about 30–60 seconds). Gently turn the tortilla and cook until side two can also easily be lifted with the spatula.

5. Repeat with the rest of the tortillas, overlapping them on a large plate rather than making one tall stack (which can soften and steam them too much).

6. If you don't have a non-stick pan, you can get good results with well-seasoned, recently oiled cast-iron skillets, but your mileage may vary.

7. Smear each tortilla with some mashed avocado, and top with some hot carnitas. Serve with sour cream, shredded cheese, and salsa, if desired.

8. Serve the chopped salad in individual bowls.

Carnitas Taco Salad

If you want to make Carnitas Taco Salad instead of tacos, skip the tortillas and stir some of the mashed avocado into a juicy serving of chopped salad to make a nice dressing for your greens. Toss your chopped salad "dressing" with your salad greens and carnitas, and if desired, top it with salsa, sour cream, and cheese.

Your tasks for this chapter:

1. Get a slow cooker – but you don't have to wait for it to start. Grab a big covered pot and get to work. All of these recipes can be made on the stovetop; you just can't leave it for the day like you can with the slow cooker.

2. Use your journal to write down the recipe ideas from this chapter or any other ideas that come to mind inspired by our suggestions. Think of a day of the week, Sunday or other, when you can prepare a large amount of food like we suggested. Make a shopping list for these meals and your other meals during the week. Cook your first meal on the chosen day, and pack up the rest. Enjoy knowing that you have two more quick and delicious dinners already planned out and ready to go!

3. Divide and conquer. If possible, shop for your ingredients ahead of time. Devote your Sunday to enjoying the cooking process.

4. Spend some time journaling about what you would like to do on the nights when you won't have to cook. Now that your fridge or freezer has the prepared meals, how would you rather spend your time? Watch a movie with the kids? Help them with homework? Finish a home project that's been waiting for months? Picture all the free time and how you would invest it – this is a great way to motivate yourself to prepare food in advance.

5. For more Sunday Food Ritual meals and their shopping lists, go to eatmovelive52.com.

Where to next?

1. Tame Your Sugar Monster (p.110)

2. In future chapters, you'll get to choose, but for now, onto Tame Your Sugar Monster

2 Grocery Wars

by Roland

Ingredient espionage and today's dietary Cold War

We are living in a new Cold War – this time it's less about bombs and more about control of our food. On one side we have the big guys – government organizations, big corporations, politicians, and lobbyists form the biggest, most well-equipped armies – with only grassroots groups, guerilla growers, and individual activists on the other side, taking a stand for the little guy. In fact, most of them *are* the little guy.

It's a tough war to wage. Like all wars, this one is full of both true stories and propaganda; there's carefully crafted news of the small farmer said to have lost a battle with a giant chemical company, epidemics are blamed on the traditional food and preparation methods of our ancestors, and government raids occur on unarmed cows who are merely minding their own business producing raw milk. Both sides spread "news" designed to make themselves look good and the other guy look bad.

Nutritional Propaganda

The biggest problem in nutrition information is not so much getting information, but identifying what information is important and what's real. Today it's all out there, but it's often coming from sources designed to seem trustworthy, even if they're not. Information comes in so fast that no one can keep up with the details, much less filter out the conflicting information. We tend to only see the headlines, and those headlines usually freak us out more than they help us out:

"Red Meat Bad"

"Toxic Sugar"

"Are GMOs Killing Us?"

"Study Finds Organic Foods No More Nutritious Than Conventional Foods"

With most of what we read in the news, the headline was written by someone who didn't write the article, and may not have even read it, much less the studies that article addresses. The headline is meant to sell papers or magazines, or to get you to click on it, even at the expense of false advertising.

It's bad enough when someone reads an article or a study and comes to the wrong conclusions, but when we only use the headlines to make decisions, we give up our power. What we're left with is restaurants, government organizations, schools, and parents making food choices that are based on headlines and not the true stories and studies behind them.

Eat better food by choosing better ingredients

Go past the headlines, and you'll still find conflicting information; one day coffee is good, the next it's bad. Red wine good, red wine bad. The same goes for things like eggs, wheat, soy, quinoa, and practically every other thing we love to eat or drink. In fact, the more "we" love something, the more it seems to be studied, fought for, and warned against.

Look, no food is perfect. Each comes with risks and rewards. Every food is filled with nutrients and anti-nutrients (yes, that's a real thing). Some foods can be great for one person, but terrible for another. Genetics, lifestyle, and health also play a big role in how your body handles food. So what's the answer? Focus on whole, unprocessed, unpackaged foods when possible.

Concentrate on "good guy" foods in their natural state, first and foremost, and when you're buying or eating something in a box, can, jar, or bag, use your spy skills to ferret out the "bad guys."

Good guys, bad guys

There are no bad foods...only there really are.

There are ingredients in our foods that prevent us from reaching our optimal health, weight, and fitness levels. You don't typically find these foods as raw ingredients in a farmer's market bin, but you do tend to find them on the ingredient labels on packages and hidden in the items on restaurant menus.

One example is man-made trans-fats, which are well-known bad guys. These partially hydrogenated vegetable oils are now being

---

Can processed and packaged foods be healthy?

Sure, but when we suggest minimizing processed and packaged foods, we're talking about highly or overly processed foods, not most basic processing or packaging that makes an ingredient safe to eat, easy to transport, or preserved for storage.

Ground beef is processed, of course. Grapes usually come in packages. Sauerkraut is both processed (chopped and fermented) and packaged (the jar). There's a wide range of packaging and processing that's perfectly acceptable, and generally understood to be so, even by the staunchest of nutritional perfectionists and body hackers.

Until we come up with different words to describe the many degrees of separation between a picked and bagged apple and a 100-ingredient, shelf-stable apple Danish, we'll have to stick with "processed" and "packaged," and you'll just have to use your head.

The danger of dismissing the advice to minimize processed foods because "everything is processed" is that you might end up winning your personal war against bad logic, but losing the war for good health.

Bad Guys

Margarine, shortening, imitation and simulated butters and spreads
Hydrogenated fats and oils, also known as trans-fats
Non-dairy creamers and sugary, calorie-rich coffee drinks
Corn oil, soybean oil, vegetable oil, and seed oils (sunflower, safflower, cottonseed, etc.)
Bottled salad dressings and dressing mixes (often contain bad oils from the above list)
Sugar, high fructose corn syrup, agave syrup, concentrated juice, and other sweeteners, no matter how natural they sound
Artificial sweeteners
Sodas and juices
Alcoholic beverages
Heavily processed packaged foods
Highly processed grains and grain-based foods
Soy products, with the exception of fermented soy products like soy sauce, miso, and tempeh
Chemicals, preservatives, and things that you can't identify, recognize, and pronounce
Deep-fried/breaded foods

MSG (monosodium glutamate), artificial colors, artificial flavor, natural flavor, and even flavors named after a real food, like strawberry flavor or chicken flavor, natural or not

E ingredients, or Es, as Europeans call them, is a numbering system for artificial ingredients, colors, preservatives, and flavorings. They are listed as a capital E and three numerals (E621, E951, etc.). Not all Es are bad (like paprika), but a lot of Es is a bad sign.

For more thorough information on the good guys and bad guys, check out our list in the resources section: eatmovelive52.com.

labeled, and sometimes even banned, with very few arguments from anyone. But despite the laws and consumer pressure to eliminate trans-fats, you might still find yourself eating a cookie filled with them if you don't read the ingredient label.

Take a look at the list of bad guy foods on these pages. Some of these are foods themselves, while others are ingredients in packaged foods. Either way, these foods are not healthy, and no amount of fish oil, vitamin pills, or superfoods can cancel them out.

Your tasks for this chapter:

Remember, the title of this week's path is Ingredient Espionage, so get your spy gear (in this case, your smartphone or tablet) ready. I have to warn you, this week's path is a thinking exercise as much as a doing exercise, but it's not that bad.

1. When you shop, look at the labels, stickers, and health claims on the box or package of everything you plan to buy, much less eat. Does the package claim to be a healthy food? Do the manufacturers use statements that suggest good health: low fat, high protein, fiber rich, or a good source of vitamins and minerals, for instance? Do the pictures on the package insinuate that the food is wholesome? Make a mental note of the claims.

2. Turn the box or package around and read the ingredient list. With any luck, the list will be short. With more luck, you'll recognize everything on it. With even more luck, the list will be nothing but natural, healthy ingredients. Unfortunately, if it's a popular, packaged food product, you'll likely find a long list of ingredients. And even if the ingredient list is short, a high percentage of them will likely be on our bad guys list. Most likely, the list of bad guys will be looooong. Two birds, one stone.

3. If the packaged food you're investigating passes muster, congratulations! Put it in the cart! Assuming you've found out the worst, it's time to look for better options or just take a pass. Most packaged foods have good (or at least better) alternatives, but if you can't find one, skip it and choose a totally different food to purchase.

You've pushed your cart through the store, reading, scanning, and spying out those bad guys, and replacing them with better choices. It might be a challenge, but this isn't forever, remember? Your current path (or mission) is about investigating foods and spying out their ingredients, and making the best choices you can, depending on what you discover.

There are no hard and fast rules; this is about awareness more than anything. As with most things, perfection is not the goal. Long term, your goal should be to find a good balance between leading a happy life and having a healthy body.

Gather your info, be a good nutrition spy, and make the best decisions you can. See how you feel about your choices at the end of this lesson. You might just find that you want to keep going.

Where to next?

1. Good Fat, Bad Fat (p.77)
2. Eat Yourself Straight (p.72)

3

Slow Down Your Meals

by Galina

From choosing to savoring your food, a snail's pace makes all the difference

Sometimes we eat, but we aren't thinking of our food. We're thinking of the past or future or mulling over some worry or anxiety again and again. So stop thinking about your business, about the office, or about anything that isn't happening right now. Don't chew your worries, your fear, or your anger. If you chew your planning and your anxiety, it's difficult to feel grateful for each piece of food. Just chew your food.
— Thich Nhat Hanh, *How to Eat*

Margie is a well-read woman in her 50s, with a couple of kids still living at home and a husband with heart disease. The whole family comes to see me for a stress management program once a week. We do some guided mindfulness work and gentle stretching and they seem to approach it with enthusiasm and gratitude.

When I ask about diet, they claim they eat very well, yet a deeper look shows that many of the salads they eat come from the cooler section of a supermarket, the chicken is from a rotisserie, lunches are squeezed between slices of whole grain bread and eaten on the go. A couple of times a week they hit an Italian restaurant ("but never have a whole pizza!").

"We do our best, we just don't have time to do more!"

"What about mealtimes?" I ask. "How long does it take you to eat?"

"We don't sit to eat," Margie admits. "Everyone kind of figures it out, I like to stand at the kitchen counter and read the newspaper while eating, Kyle crashes on the couch with a light beer, and the kids take food up to their rooms. I guess we only share popcorn on movie night."

Margie and Kyle are not the exception; they are more of a rule in our society. How many meals did your family eat together this week? If it's more than one meal every five days, you are doing better than the rest of our society and represent one of the last families keeping this tradition alive.

I remember my shock when I first visited an American family for the summer when I was 19. In Eastern Europe mealtimes are when everyone gathers at the table and shares food. Chores get dropped, homework is left for later, computers are shut down – and people just eat.

My Midwestern host family didn't once eat together throughout my visit. When I first got there, I went to bed hungry several days in a row, before one of the daughters asked me why I didn't just help myself to something from the fridge. It then dawned on me that the only time I saw them eat together was in the morning, over coffee and a bowl of cereal, which hardly qualified as food in my culture.

Slowing down to eat and really focusing on the meal and nothing but the meal has potentially huge implications for our health. On a very practical, physiological level, proper digestion requires chewing, swallowing, and significant time for satiety signals to kick in. Hormones, like CCK, GLP-1, and PYY, take 20 minutes or so to be fully released in the bloodstream after a meal. It also takes time for the body to become aware of rising levels of blood glucose. The more time you have for satiety signals to reach the brain, the more likely you are to eat an appropriate amount of food for your size and appetite. The faster you eat, and the bigger the bites, the more likely you are to over-consume energy in a short window before saticty signals have been perceived by the brain.

Speeding through a meal also robs us of noticing the colors, flavors, and aromas, appreciating the work that went into each bite, blessing the hands that prepared it, and being aware of chewing, swallowing, and fullness. Mindful eating has been shown to decrease risk of obesity, lower blood sugar, and increase satiety. Eating a meal fast has been related to increased risk of metabolic disease.

You probably know about these rules and maybe even strictly follow them, but how about speeding through the rest of your relationship with food? Do you let others prepare it, choose the ingredients, do you choose a microwave over a slow cooker or a frozen meal over a fresh one? Do you rush through the supermarket to get out of there as fast as you can? Have you completely outsourced your food preparation to a delivery company?

I invite you to think of food not just as something that needs to slow down its transit from your plate to your stomach, but also as something that has a history and life of its own, from the time you select it to the time you prepare and consume it.

I hypothesize that such an attitude can lead to a healthier relationship with what we eat and also influence how we view our bodies. It creates a more solid connection between how we perceive and treat our food and deepens the communication with our bodies through feeding behaviors.

In a world gone crazy with hurry, slow down the very thing that keeps us alive and well – our food.

Shopping

While purchasing your food, take note of how it got to the store. At the supermarket, read some labels, and choose domestic over imported. Visit the local and organic section and see what your local farmers have to offer. The longer food has travelled to get to you, the more its nutrients will have dwindled, the greater the environmental footprint it's left, and the less it will support your local economy. Often you'll find that frozen food has travelled less. There is a brand of ground beef in our local health food store that proudly states: "Meat from New Zealand, Australia and South Africa." I won't buy it – this meat has travelled from three different corners of the world to be ground and possibly mixed here in California, and that is somewhat scary.

At the farmer's market, talk to your farmers: How far do they grow from you? Did they start doing this recently or were they always farmers? How hard is it to grow kale? Are the chickens free roaming? Do they have a rooster? Becoming interested in your food is the first way to slow down your nutrition experience and to really start taking in the history, the origins and roots, and to grow an appreciation for how much work goes in each carrot, chicken egg, or bottle of olive oil. When you take those foods home and prepare them, you already have a relationship with them – they are no longer just calories, they are nourishment. You are eating the food, but also recognizing the hard work that went into producing it and making it accessible to you. This is more likely to make you appreciate and savor that carrot salad, and feel like you have had enough. The experience goes beyond chewing and swallowing, reaches beyond the taste and aromas.

Preparation – touch your food

"You need to wash your hands in the salad if you want it to taste good." The wise words of my great-grandpa, a butcher and food-lover, stay with me to this day. So do the images of Ethiopians using fingers to eat, Japanese cooks touching fish to tell its flavor, my own grandma sticking a finger into milk to see if the temperature was right for starting the yogurt. Recently, I took a course in digestive health from Barbara Loomis, a reproductive health massage therapist, and she stressed the importance of developing sensitivity to our food through touching it. "Digestion starts in the brain, not in the belly," Barbara pointed out. "Even if you are baking, move the flour from the cup into your hand." Feeling, sensing, smelling, observing, and imagining what your food can become is an important piece in reconnecting what nourishes us with our most primitive roots.

Once touched, the food informs us not only of how to treat it in preparation, but also primes our digestion for the right type and amount of digestive enzymes, as the brain recognizes which specific nutrients are going to be ingested. In this way we not only prepare our digestion so food doesn't feel like an unexpected guest popping into our stomach, but we are also starting to satiate our appetites, reaching fullness sooner. Picture touching an apple, smelling it, chopping it finely, using your hands to mix it with spices, then drizzling it with some yogurt and aromatic honey – you have just spent several minutes already eating with your hands, nose, and eyes. When you start to take the first bite, rich saliva starts to pour; abundant digestive juices are already at hard work. Compare this to driving to a window, asking for a sandwich, paying for it, and taking a bite out of a wrapper. Your brain and body have no idea what's coming or where it came from, how much of it is coming or how to know if that's enough.

The next time you make a meal, take time to touch the cucumbers for your salad, feel the juice of the lemon drip through your stinging fingers, press the meat for doneness instead of using the thermometer. Over time, your primal instincts will awaken, you will be able to tell which tomato will go in a salad, and which will make a good sauce, what spice to put in your tea for soothing a sore throat, and exactly what food can make you break the weight plateau you have reached. Opening the fridge won't feel like a puzzle, your eyes and hands will lead you to the foods you need in the moment.

Many of our clients have told us that touching food was the missing link in resolving digestive upset, bloating, overeating, or a cycle of emotional and binge eating. It has also made them better shoppers, home chefs, and more mindful and compassionate eaters.

Slow down your cooking

You may take great care to obtain local and responsibly raised and farmed food, yet completely wreck it by cooking in the fast lane. Often, you throw a great piece of steak on the grill or choose to roast your potatoes and carrots at 400 degrees, in a hurry to get them on the table in time for dinner. In recent years we have seen mounting evidence of the benefits of slow-cooked food. Several chemicals, a mouthful to pronounce, such as heterocyclic amines, polycyclic aromatic hydrocarbons, and a whole class known as advanced glycation end products, are formed through food interacting with high heat in dry roasting, direct-heat grilling, pan- or deep-frying. Those chemical reactions occur alongside the development of delicious flavors and mouth feels, such as the golden taste and irresistible crunch of a bite of well-cooked carnitas, and it's possible that we are all consuming too many of them. The fat dripping on coal creating fires of delicious smoky fumes? Great on the taste buds, but not so gentle on our DNA.

Studies link diets abundant in the chemicals produced as byproducts of cooking at high temperatures with diseases of modern life, such as obesity, type 2 diabetes, Alzheimer's, and various cancers. Instead of frying, pan searing, roasting, and grilling, why not try to steam, poach, boil, slow cook, and simmer your food? Many traditional soups, stews, tagines, goulashes, Dutch oven and hot pot meals protect food by allowing a slower preparation and deep flavor development, create nourishing broths and juices, and even take less supervision than the faster heat methods, freeing up time for you to enjoy doing something else while the meal is being prepared.

At home, our slow cooker is going all the time, either with the week's dosage of broth or a stew brewing. There is nothing better than placing some raw ingredients in the pot in the early morning, only to be welcomed home by the delicious aroma of dinner already made.

Slow down, you eat too fast

We are a fast-food nation, not just in how we obtain our food, but also in how fast we clean our plates. You may wait too long to eat, and then end up wolfing down your portions, half chewing your food. Or maybe you have a great meal plan, yet only have 5 minutes between appointments to have a cup of soup and a piece of bread.

It's really not hard to slow down, once you realize that you have been going fast. I suggest that about once a week, until you have made your meals last slightly longer, you do an eating-speed calibration exercise.

We call it "the one raisin meal." In essence, you take a raisin and sit down with it, spend some time looking at it – observing the color, the golden or brown hues, the texture of the skin, wrinkly, dry and wet at the same time. Squish it between your fingers, noticing how hard or soft it is. Bring it up to your nose, pick up smells and imagine the flavors you are about to taste. Then place it in your mouth and hold it there for a while without chewing it. Spend a minute or so, feeling the raisin in your mouth and noticing how it takes space in there, how your tongue and cheeks react to the raisin. Notice your growing desire to chew it and swallow it – tune in to this impulse and then take your first bite. Enjoy the sweet juice flowing out, find out if there are any seeds in there – how is the inside different from the outside? As you swallow, remind yourself of the power of one. Can one of anything feel like enough? I learned this exercise from Geneen Roth, who comments: "This exercise reminds us that enough is possible and it doesn't take a truckload of love to feel our hungry hearts."

Letting your meal take the space it deserves in your life is crucial to developing mindfulness. Mindful eating has been shown to decrease anxiety and depression, help with excess weight, diminish physical symptoms of discomfort, and help reduce binge eating and overeating.

Slow-mo clean up

When we teach cooking classes we often run short on clean-up volunteers. Our students love to chop, but when it's time to clean up, they are quick to scatter, pretending to be talking about something important, like the difference between a Meyer and a sweet lemon. Just yesterday, we had a very enthusiastic clean-up volunteer, David. As I congratulated him on the superb work and the shiny dishes, he said, "Oh, this is my time to be alone and do just one thing." And it's so true – dishes can turn into an opportunity to spend time in attentive awareness of the moment, learning to give the dishes the cherished recognition every aspect of our life deserves.

If while washing dishes, we think only of the cup of tea that awaits us, thus hurrying to get the dishes out of the way as if they were a nuisance, then we are not "washing the dishes to wash the dishes." ... If we can't wash the dishes, the chances are we won't be able to drink our tea either. While drinking the cup of tea, we will only be thinking of other things, barely aware of the cup in our hands. Thus we are sucked away into the future – and we are incapable of actually living one minute of life.

— Thich Nhat Hanh, *The Miracle of Mindfulness*

Your tasks for this chapter:

1. Choose one category of slo-moing your food this week – shopping, preparation, chewing, or clean-up.

2. Try the "one raisin meal." Stop by our Facebook page or send us an email to let us know how it went.

3. For a video demonstration of the raisin exercise, head over to eatmovelive52.com.

Where to next?

1. Goodbye, Turkey Head (p.181)
2. Redefine Your Core (p.215)

4 Learning to Cook from the Pros by Galina

Take your home cooking to the next level

The secret behind a good meal is the ingredients – simple and real.
— Chef Nikolay Dimitrov

Chef Nikolay, or Nicky, is the chef and owner of Sage Bistro, a lovely piece of culinary heaven nestled at the foot of Vitosha mountain in Sofia, Bulgaria. Sage is where I used to celebrate my birthdays, have long dinners with close friends, and now it has become my first destination when I land hungry at the Sofia airport.

He is someone I trust highly with my food – he is not only an inspiring professional, but he also grows a lot of his own produce in his garden and greenhouse and knows the true heart of food at its source. He is a farm to table modern hero, bridging the gap between busy lives and real food prepared simply and beautifully.

Sage Bistro just won the most prestigious restaurant of the year award in Bulgaria – a distinction well deserved! When it was time to write this chapter, I reached out to Nicky for tips and tricks to help elevate your cooking to the next level.

As a chef with years of experience, what are the big time-savers that you employ in the kitchen that could also help our readers improve their home cooking?

The biggest time saver is being prepared. Preparation means creating a shopping list that best suits what you want to make and then preparing some of the basic ingredients beforehand. There really isn't anything wrong with cooking something and freezing it. It will be much better than something you bought in the store. It saves a ton of time to have your broth cooked and frozen in bags or ice cube trays to use later in soups or sauces. You can make home-made tomato sauce and freeze that in small bags and use as appropriate. Things like lasagna or soup can hold well frozen for a long time.

What are some simple ways to elevate home cooking to restaurant levels?

The experience of eating a meal at a restaurant has so many other aspects than just the food itself. Don't forget that a restaurant has a whole team at work so that you'll enjoy your meal. At home you usually just want to eat something and get on with your evening. Sometimes it's as simple as slowing down and paying more attention to your food, but there are some simple techniques you can employ, too.

Take garlic. If you are going to use garlic in your sauce, instead of using it raw you can roast it beforehand as a way to deepen and enrich the flavors of your sauce. You can keep the roasted garlic in your fridge and add it last minute to your meal – this goes back to being prepared.

Another very simple tip is to use very high quality olive oils – if you flavor your food with higher quality oils it will be simply amazing. You can also infuse your oils with herbs and spices and create unique and very sophisticated flavors.

Using very basic ways to cook fish is one example of how great results come from small effort. People erroneously tend to think fish is hard to make. The best fish we make at Sage is one we merely bake in sea salt. We put a few herbs in the belly of the fish and then cover it with sea salt and bake.

Another simple and foolproof technique for steak and fish is to pan sear. Just place a very hot pan on the stovetop. Season your meat or fish with salt and pepper and then give it a bit of color on one side for 1–2 minutes and then the same on the other. You then transfer the pan to a hot oven. Because the meat has already been sealed from the outside, and the flavors and texture have started developing, the hot oven just finishes the process. Place the pan-seared fish on a plate and season with just balsamic and olive oil – it is excellent.

Are there any ingredients that you feel are underappreciated?

I have my favorites. Creating your own flavored oils is something that people don't realize adds a lot of character to a meal. You can make your own rosemary oil and then pour some over plain grilled chicken or pasta. You can also freeze your olive oil with the herbs inside and use it as a spread.

To add flavor to vegetables, I often use beef consommé. Peel some carrots, boil them in water and then cut them up, place them in a hot pan and add a couple of frozen cubes of consommé – beef or even vegetable stock. Flavoring them in the last few minutes of cooking in this way is really delicious.

I know you grow a lot of vegetables. Is there something that you feel is really worth growing fresh that makes a difference in the kitchen?

It depends on your skill and growing season. Sometimes I get overly excited and my greenhouse ends up looking like a jungle, but I want to utilize every space available. Even before we had the greenhouse, I had a large metal container on my balcony and grew tomatoes and corn. It's worth growing specialty salad greens, and one thing that grows like crazy is arugula. Another is mustard greens. I use both for salads and pesto.

There is nothing like a tomato that you just picked from your garden. I know that there are fancy tomatoes on the market, but they can't compare to a simple tomato you grew yourself. I prefer to use seeds from tomatoes that have been growing in my neighbors' gardens or my own. Keeping the seeds and using them the next year protects the crop from the diseases of the area – it builds a local immunity, so your plants are more robust.

Herbs are also very easy to grow. Say that you wanted to go and buy fresh-cut herbs from a store. By the time you get the herbs back to your kitchen they would not be fresh anymore. If you have good soil and a container you can grow rosemary, mint, cilantro, thyme, parsley, basil. It's really a skill accessible to anyone, and lets you reach out and pick fresh herbs at any time. You can easily give even a simple meal very different flavors every time by incorporating fresh herbs from your garden.

How do you stay in shape around all this amazing food?

You move a lot in the kitchen. I mapped my walking once on my phone and I think I got 5 miles in one evening in just a couple of hours. I never sit still or sit down to eat in the kitchen. I also eat tons of vegetables and I eat as healthy as I can. For me I think it's lots of moving and eating healthy that helps me stay in shape. It takes discipline though. We make fresh bread every day; I try not to eat a lot of the bread, and it's hard to say no.

Talking to Nicky made me feel really good about our own kitchen shortcuts. Roland and I have become good at preparing many of our staples in advance, but we have also started to simplify our meals more and more, especially when we are short on time. The result is simple, healthy, and delicious food that's better than most restaurant dishes, even if it's never going to be as good as Chef Nicky's. That's what trips back to Sage are for!

Flavored oils

Below are some of the flavored oil recipes we worked on after our conversation with Chef Nicky. Try them for yourself and take your flavors to the next level!

Herb-infused olive oil

Heat 1 cup of high quality olive oil over low heat. Place 5–6 fresh springs of rosemary and cook for about 5 minutes. Strain into a bottle. For decorative purposes you can choose to leave the rosemary inside the bottle where it will keep infusing. This oil is amazing on fish and poultry, and will enliven any pasta or rice dish.

The ingredients we always keep in our freezer for a quick dinner: broth frozen in ice cube trays, cooked rice, homemade tomato sauce, sautéed onion, cooked meatballs, and various vegetables. In the fridge we keep cheese, tortillas, various fresh vegetables, slow-cooked meat, boiled potatoes, and smoked fish. In the pantry we have rows of cans: chickpeas, green beans, lentils, pumpkin, salmon and tuna, seaweed snacks, ghee and flavored ghee, coconut milk.

Garlic-infused olive oil

Roast garlic without peeling it at 350°F for about 30 minutes. You can roast the whole bulb, or separate the cloves for shorter cooking time. Once done, peel the garlic and mix with olive oil heated on low. Infuse for 10 minutes, then drain and pour in bottles.

Chai spice–infused ghee

As a ghee addict, nothing makes me happier than seeing that I can kick my ghee-joy up a notch. To make spice-infused ghee, melt 1 cup ghee over low heat, add 5 cloves, 1 short cinnamon stick, a piece of star anise, 3 cardamom pods, 2 inches vanilla bean. Let it cook for 5 minutes, then strain and store in a jar with some extra spices – cloves and cardamom look great in there. Use to make desserts or to stir into cooked rice.

Your tasks for this chapter:

1. Think of your favorite restaurant meals. What is the quality that attracts you the most: the slow-cooked meat that falls off the bone? The crispy yet delicate veggies? The garlic dipping sauce for the bread? Try to make that at home next time. Reach out to us for the techniques you will need or consult your cookbooks.

2. Make one flavored oil and try to season simple pasta or chicken with it.

3. Plant some herbs or buy a pot of planted herbs from your local health food store or nursery.

Where to next?

1. Grocery Wars (p.15)
2. Food is Medicine (p.50)

5

Take the Soda Challenge by Galina

Refresh yourself with homemade soda

It's 2006 and I am lying in bed doing a visualization exercise. The exercise looks very much like a hypothetical movie: I enter my kitchen, thirsty, my mouth dry from the heat outside. I open the fridge. Inside I see a couple of cans of Diet Coke and a large blue-colored bottle of water. I reach for the water, open it, take a couple of satisfying sips and feel the cool liquid slide down my throat and make its way to my stomach, quenching my thirst. A smile comes to my face. I've conquered something. I've said no.

Wonder why I'm hypnotizing myself? Well, I've been dealing with a Diet Coke addiction for a while.

I don't like how I feel after I drink it, but for whatever reason, the craving keeps coming back, haunting me with its refreshing promises, taunting me to have "just a little."

It gets so bad I stock up and keep glistening cold cans at work and at home. During the day, Diet Coke is always playing sidekick to my espressos. Like a powerless addict, I go home at night, have a glass, and start dinner. Then have another glass after dinner.

The moments of opening the can or bottle, with expectations of sweetness, immediate relief, and explosive joy, have become oases in my day. On days when I've had too much, the migraines come. On other days, it's just successions of sweet cravings and poor nutrition decisions. And then sometimes, I am just too weak to say no and I drink a whole family-size bottle, consequences be damned.

Fast forward to 2007. I am able to wean myself off Coke after a few months of visualizations, disciplined decisions, and eventually learning not to buy it. Just a month off the soda helps me recalibrate and develop new habits – choosing water and sparkling water instead. When the cravings come, I invent creative recipes and quench my thirst without compromising my health.

What's wrong with soda, you may ask? Why is the US government planning to tax sugary drinks? Is this a public health myth, an urban legend, or is there really something to it?

Most of you reading this book may not remember, but soda serving sizes are much bigger now than they were 60 years ago.

"Before the 1950s, standard soft-drink bottles were 6.5 ounces. In the 1950s, soft-drink makers introduced larger sizes, including the 12-ounce can, which became widely available in 1960. By the early 1990s, 20-ounce plastic bottles became the norm. Today, plastic bottles are available in even larger sizes, such as the 1.25-liter (42-ounce) bottle introduced in 2011" (Department of Nutrition at Harvard School of Public Health).

A 6.5-ounce bottle of soda contained an average of 5 teaspoons of added sugar. A 42-ounce bottle of soda has 32 teaspoons of added sugar. The American Heart Association advises no more than 6 teaspoons of added sugars for women per day, and no more than 9 for men!

Studies on sugary drinks show links to obesity, metabolic syndrome, heart disease, and gout. We can attribute that to the sugar content, as well as the correlating habits of people who tend to choose sugary drinks regularly. For example, kids who consume more soda are also more likely to watch TV and be sedentary. That adult at the drive-through who got the double burger, fries, and Coke has more than the soda to worry about!

Studies on diet beverages seem less conclusive: Some show an effect on weight while others don't, and yet another recent study looked at how different sweeteners affect the composition of our microbiome, that complex ecosystem of bacteria that interact with the foods we consume and produce various compounds that affect our health – from our immune system to our metabolic and even

> One of my favorite clients realized he was addicted to soda and was spending as much on it as he did on an entire day's food. He gave up soda, saved over $300 a month, and lost 50 pounds... and that was the only change he made!

mental health. Is it possible that sweeteners affect our gut bacteria, which in turn affect our health outcomes? It's definitely plausible.

The body has a hard time registering calories from liquids. You may down 400 calories worth of juice and still have a full-sized breakfast. This can lead not only to systemic overconsumption of energy, but also to increased weight and increased risk for various diseases. Carbohydrate calories require a great deal of physical activity to get used, and most people are not professional athletes.

What about diet soda? We don't have sufficient scientific data to claim that sweeteners will make your nerve endings fall off and die or that they are altering your digestive system beyond repair. But people rarely analyze how drinking the diet versions of popular drinks leads to justifying other choices. Maybe they'll have an extra cookie, or those fries, but keep the diet drink. Maybe they'll succumb to the body's hunger signals when it's screaming for dessert after they've just had a full meal. The effects of diet soda may be more far-reaching than any study done so far has been able to replicate. I know that the more diet drinks I used to have, the more likely I was to crave sweets later in the day and the more calories it would take to satisfy my hunger.

Anecdotally, all of our clients and their families have found that managing the soda habit and incorporating other drinks in their daily menus, saving juice and favorite fizzy drinks for holidays and special occasions, has impacted their health tremendously.

That's why we invite you to share a challenge we do with all of our clients: Go without soda and liquid calorie drinks for two weeks. That includes all sodas – diet or regular – and juice. The goal of the exercise is to notice how you feel when you cut them out, and also to introduce some alternatives to sodas. As you develop a taste for delicious homemade refreshers, it's easy to include more of those healthy drinks, and fewer sodas and juices, once the experiment is over.

Clients come back from the soda challenge reporting amazing results – less bloating, improved digestion, clearer skin, better sleep, reduced appetite, better mood, clearer thinking. You'll have to try for yourself and track how going two weeks without sodas and juices affects you, but we have yet to meet someone who hasn't seen a positive effect.

Where do you start?

Begin by purging your fridge and pantry of sodas and juices. Invite your family to join in – it's definitely easier to do it as a team challenge.

Next, make a list of satisfying non-soda drinks:

Sparkling water – You can get basic sparkling waters at your local supermarket, or experiment with fancier versions like Perrier or S.Pellegrino, or my favorite, the German Gerolsteiner, which is rich in minerals to aid recovery after physical activity. Enjoy chilled, with ice, a slice of lime or lemon, a few sprigs of mint or basil.

Herb-infused water – You can make this easily by grabbing some basil, mint, sage, thyme, lemongrass, or whatever you have fresh in your garden. Grab a fistful of herbs, and place in a mortar. Crush with the pestle until leaves are translucent. This will unlock the aromatic oils from the leaves. Immerse in water, and keep in the fridge. Add lemon, ginger, orange slices, to spice it up.

Digestive turmeric drink, hot or cold – This is a favorite recipe of mine that I invented while dealing with a cold. Take half a fresh pineapple and place in a blender. Add 2 tbsp of turmeric powder and 1 tbsp of honey. Blend it all and then pour the mixture into ice cube trays. Once frozen, you can take one of these digestive-aiding, immune-building blocks, pour soda water or hot water on top and make a fizzy spicy drink or hot tea. The pineapple enzymes help turmeric absorb better, too!

Iced tea – You can make delicious unsweetened iced tea by simmering some rooibos tea and then chilling it in the fridge. Rooibos has a naturally deep, smoky and sweet flavor that helps with sweet cravings and satisfies even the most picky iced tea drinkers.

You can be creative and make any combination of herbs, oils, fruits, teas, still and sparkling water, from the old-fashioned spa water with cucumber slices, to fancy ginger and lemongrass-infused water. And there are lots of books out there about fruit-infused water (see the resource section at eatmovelive52.com), but start simple and explore as you go.

Your tasks for this chapter:

1. Open your journal and put in the date of the start of your soda challenge. Start by removing all soda drinks and juices from your home and workplace.

2. Think of all the places and occasions where you opt for sodas and juices, and plan what replacements you can get – even McDonald's has wonderful unsweetened iced tea.

3. Stock up on water and soda water and try one of the recipes from this chapter.

Where to next?

1. Move Like a Baby (p.207)
2. Raw, Cooked, Juiced (p.134)

6

Detox Your Pantry

Make your pantry a safe zone, and replace the bad guys with the good guys

Late-night cookies

The other day, I met with a friend who had hired me to help him lose some weight.

Dave had not been making much progress, so we looked at his food log. It was all pretty much according to plan, but several times each week one serving of packaged, grocery store, mass-produced cookies showed up on his log under "Snacks." To be honest, I was impressed that Dave was able to just eat one serving, and I told him so.

Dave looked sheepish. "I just put it in there to hold the spot."

"For what?"

"For all the cookies I actually ate," Dave said.

"More than one serving? How many?"

"I don't know," he said. "I lost count. It was pretty late. Should I just count them? I could count them out of the bag and then put down that many servings."

"Dave, I think we have a bigger problem here than accuracy," I said. "Why are you eating all those cookies at night?"

He shrugged. "Because they're there."

Nighttime snacking is a common problem. Although there's nothing special about calories eaten late at night or any other time of day, it's far more likely that any calorie eaten at night is a calorie being *over*eaten.

Our willpower is finite. At night, we're tired, and having made

44   EAT WELL, MOVE WELL, LIVE WELL

hundreds or even thousands of decisions throughout the day, our willpower is simply gone. If there's a cookie in the cupboard, we can't resist it at night, even if we've successfully resisted it all day long.

One of the most powerful things you can do for your health and weight-loss goals is to get rid of the foods that constantly tempt you. If a food calls to you from the cupboard, you're going to eat it. Maybe not today, but probably tomorrow.

Good guys, bad guys

It's hard to argue the essential "goodness" of some foods, like salmon, broccoli, and olive oil, but "bad" foods are not as clear-cut, which is why you'll see us recommend moderation and limitation vs. total elimination.

The dose is the poison, as they say. The problem today is that we are inundated, surrounded by, and constantly subjected to bad foods to the point where they have become staples in our diet, and that's quite a dose.

The pantry cleanup

The hardest part of a pantry detox is starting – just ask Dave, who tried to get me to wait a week to help him detox his pantry, so he had time to finish the cookies that were in there. It can be hard to throw away things that you love, but remember that these foods are stopping you from meeting your goals. Commit, set aside a couple of hours, and really go through your pantry and refrigerator.

Have boxes, bags, and a compost container ready for all the garbage and recycling you'll be generating. This is also a good time to clean up those old spills and throw away everything past its expiration date.

Let's get going!

Don't stress too much about the very small details. For instance, you'll see chicken on the good list; don't worry that you have chicken drumsticks. Don't wonder if chicken breasts would be better. Chicken is good…just don't go deep frying it and we're cool with you. (And chicken nuggets, definitely not good. But you know that, right? Right?)

Good (keep)

Yes, even a good food can be overconsumed, but it's unlikely with most of the good foods that you're going to focus on, and since they are so healthy, the damage isn't severe, if it's damaging at all. Keep all of these.

Fridge and freezer – meat (chicken, turkey, fish, beef, pork, lamb, etc.), eggs, fruit, fresh or frozen vegetables, potatoes, sweet potatoes, yams, corn, condiments (ketchup, mustard, salsa, etc.), plain yogurt, cottage cheese, cheese, fermented vegetables, fermented and cultured drinks like kefir and kombucha, etc.

Pantry – nuts, seeds, canned veggies, canned meat, pickles, kraut, herbs and spices, salts, olive oil, coconut oil, whole coconut milk (not the milk carton kind), palm oil, vinegar, oatmeal, dried and canned legumes, rice, unprocessed grains (not flours, breads, etc.), salsa, etc.

Bad (don't keep)

In moderation, there are few truly bad foods, but this stuff is pretty bad to have on a regular basis!

Remember that you're not getting rid of these things forever. Just give it a fair shot and see how you do.

Fridge and freezer – ice cream, frozen yogurt, soda, margarine, juice, chocolate milk, non-dairy creamer, sweetened coffee and tea drinks, etc.

Pantry – vegetable oils, seed and soybean oils, shortening, cookies, crackers, candy, cake mixes, cereal, cheap/mass-produced bread, etc.

Also, get rid of foods that *contain* any of our bad guys from the sidebar above.

On the bubble

These are foods that might fit perfectly into many healthy lifestyles, but might also be trigger foods or eaten in a way that's not healthy (for instance, popcorn is just an ingredient, but preparation is every-thing). If you slather mayo on everything, consider taking a break from it.

Refrigerator or freezer – milk, mayonnaise, commercial salad dressings, beer, etc.

Pantry – chocolate, dark chocolate, dried fruit, peanut butter, popcorn, wine, liquor, flours, sugars, etc.

Remember to look at the ingredient lists for those bad guys!

Shop and restock

Once you've tossed out the bad stuff, cleaned, scrubbed, and organized, it's time to make a list, head to the store, and restock!

It often helps to think of certain categories when making your list.

Fats for cooking – Butter, olive oil, and coconut oil are healthy staples.

Protein sources – Fish, fowl, eggs, cheese, yogurt, cottage cheese, and meats. Even cold cuts, deli meats, sausage, and bacon are healthy choices when they aren't filled with the bad guys.

Vegetables – There really aren't any bad veggies. Even potatoes only become bad when they are turned into fries or hash browns, but even these have healthy versions. Focus on greens and green veggies, like lettuce, cabbage, broccoli, zucchini, peas, and green beans, but don't get hung up on the color green, either; veggies like tomatoes, eggplant, summer squash, and cauliflower are perfectly healthy, even though they aren't green.

Snacks – The fewer snacks you have on hand, the fewer snacks you'll be tempted to eat. Still, a few healthy snacks are fine. Focus on cut-up veggies, Greek yogurt, cheese, nuts, seeds, jerky, and fresh fruit. I love frozen blueberries topped with plain yogurt!

Dressings and condiments – Special condiments can make simpler foods fun, so experiment with fancy mustards, chili sauces, salsas, tapenades, and pestos. Most bottled dressings are filled with low-quality seed and soybean oils, plus sugar or high-fructose corn syrup. Most well-stocked supermarkets will have one or two healthier versions made with olive oil, but you might have to search the natural food stores for more choices or simply make your own. Bottled dressings are a modern invention, but olive oil and vinegar have been on tables (and salads) for thousands of years.

Desserts – The best tip here is to only buy desserts when you *must* have desserts. When you do, only buy what you are going to eat at the time. Dessert leftovers rarely survive the night uneaten. Good desserts to keep around the house are fruit and yogurt.

Your tasks for this chapter:

1. Use your journal to make a list of the foods that are both beneficial to your body and are keepers. Focus on how many of them you enjoy and plan some meals focused around them.

2. Plan a day and time to do your pantry clean-up. Get some backup, like a health-minded friend or your older kids.

3. Remember to restock your kitchen with everything you need from the list above.

Where to next?

1. Explore Your Breathing (p.260)
2. Read the Small Print (p.330)

7 Food Is Medicine

by Galina

How to use herbs and spices for flavor and healing

A herb is a friend of physicians and the praise of cooks.

— Charles the Great

I grew up as a wild herb forager. I walked the woods with my parents from a very young age and some of my first memories are of gathering nettles, chamomile, yarrow, dandelion, lavender, rose hips, and various mushrooms, and making tea in the garden for my tea parties. The love of knowing about herbs and spices, but also the courage to just experiment with them, has stayed with me since.

Not everyone has this relationship with herbs and spices. When I moved to the US, I found that parsley was merely used as garnish and that most of our friends who invited us over for dinner weren't at all brave with their herbs and spices. I soon discovered that a small bundle of dill cost over $2 and organic herbs an arm and a leg at the farmer's market. I planted my first pot of herbs about a week into arriving here, and soon after found a local patch of nettles. I was home.

People often ask me the difference between an herb and a spice. It's easy to remember. In popular culture, the leaves of plants used in cooking or medicinal preparations are considered herbs, and once you dry the leaves or other parts of the plant, such as the root or seed, they are considered spices. Cilantro, when used as chopped leaves is an herb, but its seeds, which we know as coriander, are a spice.

Herbs and spices have long been part of culinary tradition and folk medicine – they have been used to support health and to act as flavors and preservatives in cooking. All ancient systems of healing – Chinese medicine, Ayurveda, Arabic medicine, Australian Aboriginal traditions – use a wide variety of herbs and spices. Hippocrates, in Ancient Greece, had over 300 different plant remedies in his protocols.

Much of that knowledge has been passed down and today the use of herbs and spices is being studied for numerous possible health benefits. For example, garlic has been widely researched as a remedy for the prevention and reversal of coronary heart disease, as well as for its ability to fight off fungus and bacterial growth. Lemongrass, gingko, flax, and ginseng are also among the plants giving lots of hope in heart disease research and degenerative diseases of the brain. Flavonoids responsible for the rich colors in herbs and spices are becoming better understood. There have been over 4,000 of them identified, and many of them have the properties to fight oxidative damage, provide immune system support, and act as anti-inflammatory and anti-tumor agents.

A lesser known beneficial side effect of using herbs and spices is their ability to increase the bioavailability of other nutrients in food and to help us enjoy food without too much salt, sugar, dressings, or condiments. A meal that is well balanced with herbs and spices provides a lot of visual appeal, but also is very palatable and decreases the need for conventional flavorings and condiments, which often bring along high levels of industrial fats and sugars. Just by adding some common and easily obtainable herbs and spices to your tea, salads, stir fries, curries, soups, and sauces, you can support your body in daily life – helping multiple systems fight off aging and disease.

I reached out to my friend Kaisa Lopes, PhD, who combines the healing power of herbs with acupuncture in her practice in Orange County, California. She tells us about her top favorite herbs and spices.

What are some herbs and spices people could use in the kitchen to maintain health and fend off disease?

Some of the heavy hitters that pack the most punch per ounce would be garlic, ginger, cinnamon, turmeric, oregano, peppermint, rosemary, thyme, dandelion, basil, and celery. You can include those at almost any meal.

What would you recommend people have as daily support if they don't have a specific condition?

Great daily support would be incorporating ginger – it's antiviral, anti-inflammatory, anti-tumor. You can make it as tea or throw a shot of it in your smoothie or juice. I think both raw and powder work really well. I would suggest raw for sore throat and digestion, but if you are looking for more of a long-term buildup in the system, dry ginger will give you a higher dose. It's even something that you could supplement with.

Garlic is my next favorite – it's a strong antimicrobial agent. Americans can greatly benefit from this plant, because our guts are so out of balance. Garlic can be a great regulator of nasty yeast and bacteria. It's amazing for the cardiovascular system, and it's also great in the form of tea if you are coming down with a cold or the flu. I think it tastes really great. Garlic is so accessible and cheap.

My third recommendation is to add cinnamon to your food. In Chinese medicine cinnamon is used in many formulas. Cinnamon is great for lowering blood sugar, regulating bloating or gas, we also use it as a blood invigorator. Any situation in which circulation is poor – from menstrual cramps to varicose veins and cardiovascular issues. Again, you can incorporate it in your diet, and for some conditions you may need the supplement form.

Cinnamon is very popular, but many Westerners think of it as something for dessert only. How can people add cinnamon to their day?

In Latin America cinnamon is a part of tea and coffee and it's an easy way to add it to what you are already drinking. Your yogurt, your oatmeal, or your coffee are all options to add cinnamon.

My other favorite is turmeric, which has anti-inflammatory properties. Raw it's not cheap and most of my patients are not too crazy about the flavor of the raw root. We know that you need quite a bit of turmeric to get the benefits. It's amazing to cook with it in powder form and also in some cases take it as a supplement. Research shows that black pepper has a synergistic effect with turmeric, and it's easier to absorb and reap the benefits if you use them together in a recipe.

What are some green herbs that you use in your own kitchen?

My top favorite greens are parsley, oregano, and thyme. Peppermint can also be amazing with PMS, bloating, and liver cleansing. Freshness is key. By the time you buy and take herbs into your kitchen they are not that fresh anymore, so the ideal situation is "if you are not growing them you are getting them from your neighbor."

I also greatly support the use of herbs and spices in the form of essential oils. To extract the oil from a plant is an intense process and the oil ends up as an extremely potent remedy. I encourage people who want to use herbs in potent forms such as supplements or oils to consult with an herbologist to know which the best method is.

Below you will find some commonly used herbs, as well as some guidance for their use and benefits.

Parsley – Flat leaf or curly, this is our favorite herb to add to chopped cucumber and tomato salad, but also great on its own in tabbouleh salad. You can add it chopped to steamed or sautéed veggies, or use it to top stews and soups before serving.

Benefits: improves blood pressure and fluid balance, strengthens bones and the nervous system

Dill – Underappreciated in the US, dill is a main ingredient in yogurt sauces and dips in the Mediterranean. Maybe you already love dill pickles – just add dill to your cucumber salads for a fresher version of the same powerful crunch! Remember to use it with fish, potatoes, as well as with any dish that has yogurt as a base.

Benefits: Dill, like garlic, has antibacterial properties; it's been studied for its positive effects on the bones.

Coriander (cilantro) — Familiar to Mexican-food lovers, cilantro is not only an amazing topping for tacos and tortilla soup, but it also makes a great marinade or main sauce. Try it both in vegetable and fruit salsas. Pork and fish go great with it.

Benefits: blood sugar regulation, cholesterol lowering, anti-aging

Mint – This herb is equally popular in culinary recipes and as an ingredient in medicinal teas. When cooking you can add mint to salads, especially the ones including cucumbers, carrots, yogurt, or crème fraiche. It's great with cooked vegetables, chicken, and turkey, as an ingredient in ice cream, chocolate desserts, and for making ice water even more refreshing.

Benefits: improves digestion, alleviates colds and flu, fights depression, improves mood

Basil – This is tomato's best friend. Basil is amazing in all dishes calling for fresh or cooked tomatoes and sprinkled on top of any Italian meal makes it absolutely complete. The two main kinds of basil, Genovese and Thai, are used best in their respective cuisines – use Genovese for mozzarella and tomato salad, Thai for your coconut curry.

Benefits: anti-aging, anti-cancer, bone health, antibacterial, heart health

Oregano – We use two kinds of oregano – Greek and Mexican. Each has a distinct flavor and goes with Mediterranean or Mexican dishes. Raw oregano is a very easy-to-grow, potent little herb and will make any fresh veggie salad a new and unique dish. Almost any meat combines successfully with oregano, especially in slow-cooked dishes. We also like to add it to tomato dishes, lemon potatoes, risottos, and recipes with eggs and cheese. Fresh or dried oregano also makes a delicious tea.

Benefits: antiviral and antibacterial, helps symptoms of colds and flu, anti-aging

Sage – This underappreciated herb is known as "garden tea" where I come from and makes both amazing teas and enticing dishes. It's great with beef and pork, as stuffing for turkey, and to flavor soups and broths.

Benefits: memory enhancing, bone health, anti-aging, helps breathing

Rosemary – This wiry herb is not just for fancy chicken skewers. It flavors any meat perfectly, especially lamb. It goes great with slow-roasted vegetables of any kind and makes delicious tea – hot or cold. Marinating with rosemary is one of the ways to decrease the formation of harmful chemicals in higher heat cooking.

Benefits: detoxification, immune system health, digestion

Celery – Celery has powerful large green leaves and woody, crunchy stalks that make it great in salads, but also very suitable in stews and soups. Steamed celery with some lemon pepper and lemon juice is a lovely side dish.

Benefits: diuretic, digestive support, anti-oxidant, anti-inflammatory

Garlic – Both green and mature garlic are a part of many cuisines, from Asian to Mediterranean. You can use garlic in everything from sauces to soups, stir-fries, and slow-cooked meals. You can even just roast it and use it as a spread. In *Eating on the Wild Side* Jo Robinson tells about Native Americans who gathered over 100 kinds of alliums (the garlic and onion family) for food and medicine. Allicin, the active ingredient in garlic, is best released if you peel and chop the garlic and wait for 10 minutes before using it – then you can cook it or use raw.

Benefits: antiviral and antifungal, strengthens the immune system, anti-cancer, and protection from heart disease

Ginger – The rhizome is used in many Asian recipes, and as an ingredient in desserts and cookies. Think pumpkin spice – it's easy to recognize the spicy bite of ginger on your tongue and the back of your throat, both sweet and hot! Ginger can be used in smoothies and teas, as flavoring for lemonade, and to make homemade crystallized ginger – you can't beat homemade candy!

Benefits: digestion, morning sickness, immune system support, detoxification, anti-cancer

Cinnamon – There are two main types of cinnamon – Ceylon and Cassia. Most cinnamon sold in the US is the hard bark known as Cassia. Ceylon cinnamon comes in a more brittle stick and has a finer and sweeter aroma. They have quite different tastes. We enjoy cinnamon in plain oatmeal with some vanilla and ghee melted on top. Cinnamon is also great on yogurt parfaits and in most conventional desserts and baked goods. Ready for something different? You can add it to dips and sauces, as well as chili, stew, and ground meat recipes such as meatballs and Greek moussaka.

Benefits: blood pressure regulation, antibacterial and antifungal, digestive support, mood elevator, anti-cancer

Turmeric – This is the yellow spice that gives curry its deep golden color. It's a rhizome that looks like tiny ginger roots. You can include turmeric in all your cooking, from soups to stews, desserts, warm and cold drinks.

Benefits: anti-inflammatory, anti-oxidant

Cardamom – The green pods hide small seeds that you can take out and grind into a fine powder. It's amazing in tea and coffee, as an ingredient in desserts and ice creams. Cardamom mixes well with cream and milk, and is a lovely spice to add to a warm glass of milk before bed.

Benefits: blood sugar regulation, improved circulation, digestive system health, reproductive and urinary system health

Cumin – The seeds of cumin can be used both whole and ground in flavoring vegetable dishes and meat dishes. It adds amazing flavor to all ground meats, meatballs and meatloaf, as well as savory baked goods. It's also our favorite spice in homemade sausages and jerky.

Benefits: digestive support, immune system health, antiviral, and antimicrobial

Black pepper – The small seeds can be used whole or ground in vegetable and meat dishes, sauces, and as a tea. If you remember from the interview, black pepper also improves the absorption of turmeric.

Benefits: improves digestion, anti-inflammatory, anti-oxidant

Chili peppers – These little guys can be used in Mexican, Thai, or Indian food, or just to add some kick to any dish. Add them to soups, stews, salsas and sauces (like mole), and even homemade chocolate desserts.

Benefits: anti-inflammatory, pain relief, improved circulation, anti-cancer, immune system support

Your tasks for this chapter:

1. Pick up a couple of fresh herbs or new spices from the store. Specialty spice stores will by far have the best quality spices, as the ones in supermarkets tend to stay on the shelf a long time. Just do the best you can with the quality. If you're not sure what to get, go for Dr. Lopes's favorites: ginger, garlic, and cinnamon.

2. Try at least one new recipe this week that has plenty of ginger, garlic, or fresh spices. Most curries and soups are easy to make.

3. Can you add spices to your drinks? Cinnamon in your latte? Mint in your lemonade? Go for it!

4. Plan to have a couple of pots or boxes of fresh herbs on your patio or in your yard. Certain ones, like rosemary and basil, mint and thyme, are really easy to grow.

Where to next?

1. Get Dirty (p.395)
2. Quiet Time (p.268)

Eat Your Water

by Roland

8

Why you're probably not dehydrated, but still not drinking enough water

Seventy-five percent of Americans are chronically dehydrated!"... says that email your mom just forwarded, urging you to drink your "eight by eight," or 8 ounces of water, eight times per day, lest something terrible happen.

Mom, do you remember when I was a kid? What about when you were a kid? How neither of us drank our eight by eight, but *weren't* dehydrated?

I fondly remember my childhood days, when my friends and I would go all day without drinking any water at all until we were thirsty. Only then would we start looking for a house with a garden hose out front.

Water mythology

That admonishment to drink eight glasses of water each day has been floating around for so many years that it's generally accepted as true *and* good advice – but is it?

I've asked experts and done my own digging. While I found a lot of studies on the benefits of drinking enough water, there seems to be no evidence that we are chronically dehydrated. There doesn't seem to be any evidence that we aren't, either. Hmm.

Paul Ingraham is a prolific and well-respected science writer and journalist. When he investigated the problem of chronic dehydration, and whether it even exists, he found nothing. "I am unable to find any scientific research which either supports or contradicts the claim," wrote Paul in a recent *Pain Science* article, "Water Fever and the Fear of Chronic Dehydration."

I'll chalk this one up to mythology, but as you know, it's also spawned quite a few little baby myths.

"Drink your eight by eight"

Back in the 1940s, people were advised by the Food and Nutrition Board of the National Research Council that we needed to ingest about 2.5 liters of water (or about eight 8-ounce glasses) to keep ourselves hydrated, but apparently no one remembered to read to the third sentence, where we were told that we already get most of that through the food we eat:

"A suitable allowance of water for adults is 2.5 liters daily in most instances. An ordinary standard for diverse persons is 1 milliliter for each calorie of food. Most of this quantity is contained in prepared foods" (Food and Nutrition Board, National Academy of Sciences, 1945).

Of course, fruits and vegetables are mostly water, but the salty snacks, breads, and pastries populating our pantries these days are mostly dry – worth taking into account as you figure out your body's water needs.

That appears to be the first time these numbers appeared in any official recommendations, although similar numbers appeared in the writings of doctors and scientists of the day, often along with permission to count coffee, tea, and other liquids as water.

"By the time you're thirsty, it's already too late!"

There are variations on this one, but they all suggest that we don't know when we're thirsty, and have to rely on a phone app, food logs, and checkboxes to know when we've had enough to drink. However, a 2013 study in *Proceedings of the National Academy of Sciences* seems to confirm that we actually do know when we're thirsty and when we're not. The study found that our swallowing reflex is heightened when we need to drink, and it calms back down when we don't. In fact, our brains are so in tune with our bodies, the study found, that our pleasure centers are stimulated by drinking when we need it, and turned off when we don't. Yeah, we know when we're thirsty!

Are there people who don't recognize thirst? Sure, but it's fairly rare outside of hospitals, elder care, and nursing home facilities. Unless you're sick, your mind/body connection is probably strong enough to tell you when you're thirsty. So drink up…or don't!

"You're not hungry, you're probably just thirsty!"

I suppose there's something to this one, even though it's not technically true. Even though you can't forever drink away your hunger (because water isn't food), you can use a drink of water to help you get through a hungry period.

"You're not losing weight because you're not drinking enough water!"

This is one of the confusing ones. On one hand, the amount of water you drink really has nothing to do with weight loss. On the other hand, it's true that people who drink more water tend to lose more weight. So now what?

DO COFFEE, TEA, JUICE, AND ALCOHOL COUNT AS WATER?

Coffee and tea do count toward your daily fluid consumption. Even caffeinated drinks count, as caffeine is only a diuretic in large, medicinal doses. Really, all liquids count, although you take the good with the bad. Caffeine might keep you awake, but it won't dehydrate you. There's nothing inherently bad in coffee, tea, or herbal tea, so count it toward your water.

When it comes to soda, juice, and alcoholic drinks, the downsides (sugar and alcohol) outweigh the good. My general rule is to stick to drinks that have few or zero calories, and you'll be fine.

CAN YOU DRINK TOO MUCH WATER?

Technically, yes, but it's very rare and you almost have to try!

Every year or so, someone decides to have a water-drinking contest, and they end up dying from water intoxication, a condition caused by drinking water until the blood has been dangerously diluted of electrolytes! In the process of drinking a lot of water quickly, they flush out sodium and other electrolytes until levels are dangerously low.

Marathon runners and long-distance athletes can also overdrink, albeit with the best of intentions, trying to fend off dehydration. If you're an endurance athlete, or training like one, it's important to work with a qualified coach who can teach you about proper hydration and electrolyte balance before, during, and after events. When it comes to marathon events, just drinking plenty of water is not good enough.

If you're on a diet, extra water can actually help in a few ways. As mentioned, it can tide you over until your next meal. A study in the journal *Obesity* found that drinking two glasses of water before meals led to eating less without even trying. Those who drank a 16-ounce bottle of water before each meal lost weight 44% faster, and were an additional five pounds lighter at the end of the twelve-week study. It helps to pass the time, gives you something to put in your mouth, and gets you moving by making you go to the bathroom more.

Some people swear that drinking cold water forces your body to burn extra calories to warm up again. While this is true, it only adds up to about 50 calories per day. *Only* 50 calories per day. That's not much. It's like skipping seven almonds. Seven.

While the *amount* that you drink isn't doing much to help your weight loss, strategic timing of your water drinking could help. In fact, drinking a pint of water before you eat has been found to spontaneously reduce calorie intake by nearly 100 calories! That's per meal, by the way, so over the course of a day, you might end up eating hundreds of calories less than you would have without the water.

Your tasks for this chapter:

1. Check for symptoms of dehydration. Mild dehydration isn't always easy to spot, but symptoms include: thirst, dry mouth, fatigue, decreased urine output, darkened urine, dry skin, headaches, dizziness, constipation, and lack of tears when crying. Obviously some of these signs are pretty vague, so make a note and keep track of what and when you feel these things.

2. Being thirsty every once in a while is probably nothing to sweat, but if it's chronic, then…well, that's the chronic dehydration that the rest of us don't have. You better take care of it!

3. Track water intake. I know I said that we don't need to rely on food logs and apps to know when we need to drink, but not being dehydrated and being optimally hydrated are two different things. We've survived for a long time on our instincts, but that doesn't mean we can't do better.

4. If you're already using an app or program to track food, then there's a good chance that your tool has a water tracking function. I use the FitBit app, and there's a button to push every time I drink another glass. It's pretty easy in an app, but even without one, all it takes is opening a memo on your phone or jotting it down on a piece of paper that you keep in your pocket.

5. Adjust water intake. If you show signs of dehydration, then adjust your fluid levels up! The easiest way to get more fluids is to drink more fluids, obviously, but if you're not eating enough fruits and vegetables, that's a great (and healthy) way to get in more fluids. Use the table at the top of the next page to help.

90-100% water	Water, tea, coffee, broth, clear soup, cucumber, cooked squash, cooked cabbage, bamboo shoots, lettuce, celery, radish, tomato, pumpkin, spinach, tomato, canned green beans, melon, asparagus, pickles, rhubarb, turnips, rhubarb, cooked broccoli, carrots, cooked cauliflower, chard, onions, peppers, cooked kale
80-90% water	Kale, okra, mushrooms, strawberries, leeks, onions, fennel, hearts of palm, cooked eggplant, cooked winter squash, citrus, peach, artichoke, yogurt, cooked rice, cooked potatoes
50-70% water	Cooked meats – chicken, beef, pork, cold cuts, most cheeses, cooked grains
30-50% water	Dried fruits and vegetables, spreadable fats, some cheeses, dry heat cooked potatoes
15-30% water	Most baked goods, some flours, dried vegetables, dried fruits
Under 15%	Liquid fats, salt, sugar, flours, nuts and nut butters, dried meats

6. Repeat – Go back to the top and check for signs of dehydration, log your water, and adjust when necessary. You shouldn't have to do this forever, because after a few weeks, this should become habit. Still, don't be afraid to check yourself every few months, just to be sure the habit has stuck!

Where to next?

1. Just Look, You Don't Have to Touch (p.142)
2. Furniture Minimalism (p.300)

9 Take the Eating-In Challenge by Roland

A good cookbook is better than any diet book

Growing up, I cooked for my family once a week, but my version of cooking meant browning hamburger meat to stir into jarred pasta sauce.

When I started working, I began to spend my hard-earned money on fast food, restaurant meals, and salty snacks. My weight, never fully under my control, shot up without mercy. One day, I stepped on my mother's scale, and saw it stop spinning at 265. I vowed never to see a higher number on the scale…so I stopped weighing myself, and kept on eating.

When I eventually moved into my own place, I unpacked all the pots, pans, and spices I'd quietly "borrowed" from my mom, decorated the countertops with a ridiculous knife block and a huge food processor, and then walked to Arby's for dinner.

A few weeks later, I weighed myself again, and I was 275 pounds. An all-time high.

A few days after that, on my way home from yet another trip to Arby's, I took a different way home…through the grocery store.

After filling my cart with all my favorite processed foods (ramen soup, mac and cheese, hot dogs, frozen burritos, ravioli, and canned beef stew), I made a detour to the produce section just to get some bananas. In front of the fruit section was a display of Sunset Magazine Cookbooks, a straightforward little series with great pictures. The picture on the front of *Southwestern Cooking* looked good, so I picked it up. I read a few recipes right there in the produce section, picked out the simplest one, cruised back through the store to pick up the ingredients to make chili colorado (a Mexican dish of slowly cooked beef, simmering in a savory red sauce), and headed home.

The next day was Sunday, and I simmered my beef roast while I watched television. That night at dinner, I was amazed! It was the best thing I'd ever cooked. So good that I ate close to a pound of it!

Unfortunately, I'd purchased a seven-pound roast; I now had over a week's worth of meat, less if I also ate it for lunch, breakfast, and snacks. So I flipped through the book, making a shopping list inspired by the pictures: rice, tortillas, cheese, beans, broth, lettuce, peppers, and onions. To survive a week of this one-meat-experience, I had to get creative. Over the next four days, I had tacos, taco salads, shredded beef with grilled peppers and onions, a burrito that fell apart when I picked it up, and even soup!

At the end of the week, without knowing how, I'd regained one whole belt notch. Excited, I stepped on the scale, and found that I'd lost four whole pounds...without doing anything other than cook my own food.

The true cost of processed food

Processed food is cheap; even eating out can be cheap when you buy from the fast-food value menus.

Unfortunately, because of the low costs of packaged and prepared foods, and today's tendency to fill our days with soccer practices, video games, and television, people are just not cooking, and it's taking a toll on our health and waistlines more than it is on our wallets.

Each meal eaten out:

- increases calorie intake by approximately 134 calories over a meal eaten at home

- reduces fruit and vegetable serving consumption by over 22%

- reduces whole fruit consumption by over 32%

- reduces consumption of dark green and orange vegetables by 31%

- decreases dietary quality by two points on the Healthy Eating Index (HEI), enough to drop the consumer from Fair to Poor

These things add up quickly. The more meals you eat out or from a box, the more extra calories you consume, the less nutrition you get in exchange, and the more weight you tend to gain, even as nutrition from vitamins, minerals, and high-quality protein, fats, and carbohydrates plummets.

The solution is really simpler than you'd imagine: cook and eat at home.

Cook at home tips

- Use cookbooks if you need ideas. Most people have several cookbooks already, so start with what you have. If not, pick one up at your grocery store or bookstore.

- Remember to pack your lunches, too. There's no need to reinvent the wheel, simple sack lunches are fine. You can also have leftovers from last night's dinner.

- Stick to the spirit of your mission and don't look for loopholes – jars of salsa, frozen veggies, canned tomatoes, nice pasta sauces, and canned beans are fine. Frozen dinners, canned stew, and microwave pizzas are not fine.

- Remember to shop ahead and buy enough food. You don't want to drive through for fast food on the way home just because you're out of fresh food. If you don't have food to cook at home, go simple: chicken and veggies, and make your plan for tomorrow as you eat it.

- Think ahead, plan ahead, make your menus, count your meals, make your shopping lists, and go!

Your tasks for this chapter:

1. Open your journal and write down the usual number of meals eaten out or picked up every week. Write down the cost for the week. If you can't remember, then during this next week, just log your expenses – everything from coffee and a bagel at the breakfast bar at work to picking up wings for the kids. Look at your week's expenses. Now multiply that by 4 to see what it looks like each month. If the number is considerable, you may consider doing our cooking at home challenge for more than just this week.

2. Try making a recipe that will give you several days' worth of meals. (See suggestions in the resources section at eatmovelive52.com.)

3. Decide how many meals you will eat out each week on your own and with the family and stick to it for a month. Notice how that affects your digestion, weight and mood, and your wallet.

Where to next?

1. Slow Down Your Meals (p.22)
2. Learning to Cook from the Pros (p.31)

NUTRITION

10

Eat Yourself Straight by Galina

...and get better digestion in the end

Most health seekers these days are crazy smart about nutrition, but many people who reach out to us still struggle with digestive upset, constipation, extra weight, and even shortness of breath, anxiety, or fatigue after meals.

There is a lot going on between the time you select your meal to the time you get to extract energy from it, and the devil is in the details. How you sit, how you swallow, and even how much attention you pay to the process of nourishing yourself all play a part in how your body deals with your food.

The very moment you think about your dinner or look at a piece of cheesecake, your body is already preparing for digestion. Juices start flowing, peristalsis (the muscle contractions in your digestive tract) is stimulated, and your cells are getting ready to get nourished. The second you put a bite between your teeth, your chewing starts to break the food down into smaller pieces and mix it with saliva for digestion. The process of food assimilation begins in your mouth, where enzymes start to work before moving on to the stomach and down to the intestines.

This initial process is critical, and while it's not as simple as the "chew each bite 30 times" that Grandma insisted on, making sure your food is well mashed and mixed with saliva before you swallow is truly the first step to great digestion.

The next step is swallowing. Your swallowing muscles are housed in your neck and positioned for action so that the food can pass through with the least effort. In order for them to work well, your head and neck need to be in their natural alignment – head over shoulders and chin level with the floor. If your head juts forward or leans to one side, then each swallowing action gets assisted by muscles in your face and neck. This may result in tight muscles in the jaw and shoulders, higher stress levels, and eventual changes in the function of all systems in the body, affecting your muscular, endocrine, cardiovascular, and digestive systems. How your head is positioned for swallowing and breathing really matters. Try telling your chiropractor that the next time they say they don't know why your neck is out of alignment!

Chew, swallow, breathe

Have you ever been tired or out of breath after your meal? Did you ever need a nap right after eating? You may not be breathing optimally between your bites. Very much like the suck, swallow, breathe reflex of nursing babies, your chew, swallow, breathe eating pattern is an integral part of the normal physiology of the body. Depending on how you do it, you can chew, swallow, and breathe with more or less effort. Having your neck kinked and your air passage restricted when eating takes a toll on your system, but with a little practice, it's preventable.

Let's do an exercise together. Place your head over your shoulders so that the ear is right over the center of the shoulder, on each side. This head-over-shoulders alignment is optimal for swallowing and breathing.

Take a breath and let it out. Now swallow. Remember how these actions feel.

Now, jut your head forward and take a breath. Let it out. Swallow. Notice how swallowing and breathing feels very different from when you were optimally aligned for it?

Go back to proper alignment (head over shoulders) one more time, and breathe and swallow again, just to be sure.

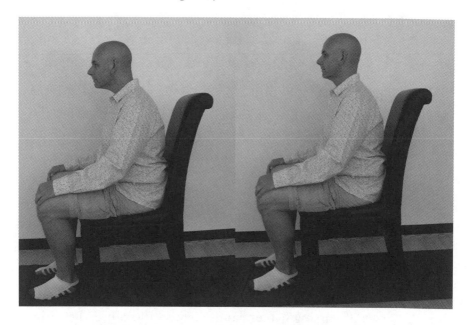

While we are on the subject of alignment, remember how your mother used to tell you not to slouch at the dinner table? Well, she was right. Having your ribcage properly positioned over the pelvis is another way to be a more efficient machine. Better alignment of the upper body provides more internal space for breathing, less compression of the stomach and intestines, and fewer kinks, twists, and turns for your breath and food to travel through. In fact, it's typically easier to eat standing up, but you can properly position your pelvis and ribcage well for sitting in just a few simple steps. Here's how:

Sit in your chair, placing the bulk of your gluteal muscles (your bootie muscles) behind you. Your pelvis will now be straight up, with the bottom pelvic bones touching the chair and your tailbone behind you. The low back will be resting in its natural curve and the upper back will be well supported. Compare this to rolling the pelvis back, sitting on the tailbone and slouching – notice the difference?

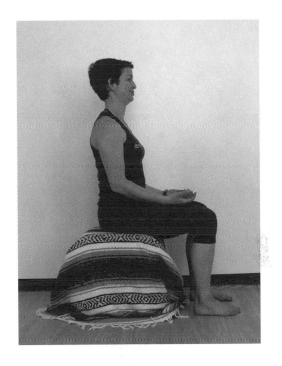

There! Your body is now well positioned for the delicious portion of your day.

Your tasks for this chapter:

1. During your meals, sit or stand up straight, paying special attention to keeping your head aligned over your shoulders.

2. Don't sit back on your tailbone, slouch, or eat quickly.

3. Keep your head aligned over your shoulders, your ribcage over your pelvis, and chew your food thoroughly.

Where to next?

1. Stand Up For Yourself (p.273)
2. Meditate on This (p.340)

Good Fat, Bad Fat

11

Cooking fats and eating fats, there's always a right fat for the right job

In the early 20th century, scientists and doctors mistakenly targeted saturated fat as the bad guy of heart health.

Almost overnight, butter and lard got a bad rap, as did meat, eggs, and any food containing animal fat. Today, we see more and more evidence that the scientists back then were wrong. Rather than continue to blame the fats, most experts are now blaming the items that typically surround these fats: the buns, the unhealthy side orders, the sugary drinks, and even the less active lifestyles of the people who tend to eat meals rich in saturated fats.

So if saturated fat is not the bad guy, why is it that some studies continue to show that people who eat less saturated fat tend to be healthier?

The healthy user bias

In the health and fitness industry, there is a phenomenon known as the healthy user bias. This simply means that people who seek to be healthy tend to do the things that they believe to be healthier, and by and large, they get it right. If they get enough of these lifestyle choices right, they end up healthier, even if some of the individual changes actually have little or no effect.

In the case of saturated fat, once word got out that it was bad, people interested in health stopped eating it as often. But those health-conscious people also tend to drink less alcohol, get better sleep, take vacations, exercise, and avoid overconsumption of treats, all of which makes them healthier, whether they cut out saturated fat or not.

NUTRITION   77

This type of bias isn't limited to eating, either. We know that exercise, activity, good work habits, good sleep, community, and many more factors affect our health. Get enough right, and your health skyrockets, even if you live a little in some areas. You don't have to be perfect to be healthy!

When it comes to saturated fat, we need to look at those other things that the healthy eaters are eating and doing to get the bigger picture.

Still, if saturated fat isn't bad, but people avoiding it are healthy, what's the problem?

Well, it turns out that the healthy eaters are still healthy, but the rest of us aren't, largely because of what replaced all that saturated fat.

What happened?

As saturated fats were left behind, they were generally replaced with polyunsaturated fats (corn, soybean, and canola oils), which are very inexpensive to produce. Monounsaturated fats (a healthy fat found in olive oil and peanut oil) also took the place of some animal fats, but because of their higher cost, their use was more limited.

Since this shift away from animal fats and other saturated fats occurred, we haven't seen a miraculous eradication of heart disease. Instead, we've seen various metabolic diseases and obesity increase, and we're only now starting to understand why.

I'm sure you've heard of the omega fats, specific types of polyunsaturated fat. Omega-3 and omega-6 are the most commonly talked about, and the most important two to consider. We can't make them ourselves, but we really need them, and we have to get them through food. Naturally, omega-3s would be found in fish and vegetables, and omega-6s in nuts, seeds, and vegetables. As we added more industrially produced polyunsaturated fats in the place of saturated fats, we also started consuming more omega-6 fats.

Historically speaking, most humans didn't consume large amounts of omega-3s and omega-6s, and when they did, they came in the form of whole foods – think fish and walnuts. Because those omega-3 and 6 rich foods weren't available in large amounts, our bodies learned to thrive on a delicate balance between 3s and 6s. Without modern farming and food manufacturing, it would have been hard to eat a lot of omega-6 fats. Nowadays our food supply is flooded with products made with soybean oil, corn oil, and canola oil. These are all fats rich in omega-6s and low in omega-3s. In addition to too many omega-6–rich foods, our society has gotten out of the habit of eating foods rich in omega-3 fats, like salmon, sardines, and herring, and when we do, we often leave the healthiest parts, like the skin, on the plate. The delicate balance of 3s and 6s has shifted faster than anyone had expected. Chronic low-level inflammation has become prevalent and has brought about the increase of many modern diseases.

In a nutshell, our bodies process omega-3s and use them to reduce inflammation. Unfortunately, omega-6s compete for the same conversion enzymes in the body, and since we eat far more 6s than 3s, the 3s lose out, and not enough get converted into a form usable by the body. Inflammation rises and stays high. Over time, this chronic inflammation leads to a variety of health conditions, such as heart disease, joint pain, asthma, arthritis, and even immune system deficiencies and psychiatric disorders.

As you can see, losing the saturated fat wasn't really the problem; what replaced it (soybean, canola, corn, and vegetable oil) was.

But wait, there's more

Too many omega-6s would be bad enough, but when food manufactures left behind saturated fats, it wasn't as simple as swapping butter for soybean oil. Butter was solid at room temperature, and was spread on foods for taste and texture. Lard made baked goods moist and even shelf stable.

With saturated fats off the menu, manufacturers had to respond, and they quickly did, by turning liquid vegetable oils solid using a process called partial hydrogenation. This process created trans-fats, by converting unsaturated fats to saturated fats, which is what we were avoiding in the first place.

Because of public pressure to remove these unhealthy trans-fats, food manufacturers eventually responded, so there *are* fewer foods with trans-fats on shelves, and the foods that still have them do have less of them. But even some of the foods proudly proclaiming themselves trans-fat free still have them because of labeling laws and loopholes that allow foods with small amounts to be labeled as zero. Unfortunately, small amounts add up quickly, and even small amounts of trans-fats are bad for your health.

Real food solves half the problem

...and the other half is easy.

Good news! If you cook at home regularly, make plenty of the food yourself, keep one eye on the ingredient lists and menus, and ask the occasional question of your server, minimizing sources of troublesome fats (omega-6s) is pretty easy. Once you're of the mindset that you're in control of your health via what goes into your mouth, getting healthy sources of fat (like monounsaturated fats and omega-3s) *into* your diet is easy, too!

Ingredient lists

First, scan the ingredient list, not the nutrition label, for fats such as soybean, corn, canola, vegetable, cottonseed, sunflower, safflower, or rapeseed oils, plus partially hydrogenated oils and fats or shortening or margarine.

Then look at the nutrition label, which will tell you how much of that fat is contained in a serving. If it's a tiny amount, like 1 gram, you may have nothing to worry about for an occasional meal or treat, but you don't want to consume those daily.

Technically, coconut, peanut, olive, and avocado oils are vegetable oils, but they tend to be healthy fats, so there's no need to avoid them.

Eating out

If you minimize your restaurant meals, then worrying exactly what's in them becomes less important. If you eat out every day, or multiple times per day, then it's really worth looking closely at the ingredient lists.

Tips when eating out

- Ask the server what oils and fats are being served and used for frying and sautéing, and ask if you can substitute healthier fats whenever possible.
- When in doubt, ask for steamed veggies and meat grilled without cooking fat.

Healthy fats for cooking

When it comes to cooking, you want to consider the taste of the fat and the cooking method.

High heat requires a fat that won't smoke easily when heated, such as avocado oil, ghee, peanut oil, or coconut oil, which have higher smoke points. Sautéing uses less heat, where olive oil, bacon fat, and butter really shine.

If you're baking, you might require a fat that's more solid at room temperature. In this case, consider using butter or lard. If being solid is not necessary, then a fat with a complimentary taste should be chosen. Light olive oil and expeller-pressed coconut oil are both relatively tasteless oils that can be used in baking when liquid fats are fine.

Fats for dressings and spreads

Choose a healthy fat that has a pleasant flavor, aroma, and mouth feel. If you're watching your calories, note that all fats have basically the same amount, so if you can find one with a stronger flavor that will allow you to use less of it, all the better.

Extra virgin olive oil is a great choice for veggies and dressings because of its distinctive taste. Creamy butter is great melted on hot vegetables. A dash of sesame oil is a lovely accompaniment to Asian dishes.

Fat as food

Many nourishing foods contain large amounts of fat, even though we don't think of them as fat. Nuts, seeds, eggs, coconut, avocados, olives, cheese, and fatty fish are great examples of healthy fat sources in whole foods.

Nuts and seeds – Although I do want you to minimize oils and fats extracted from seeds, it's very hard to overdose on omega-6s from eating the seeds themselves when you control serving sizes. In addition, the whole nuts and seeds contain many beneficial nutrients, so worrying about eating whole nuts and seeds because of the omega-6 fat isn't necessary.

Fish and fish oil – As I said earlier, in addition to minimizing omega-6s, getting enough omega-3s is important to combat inflammation. Salmon, herring, mackerel, anchovies, and sardines are great additions to your diet because they are a complete, natural source of EPA and DHA, which are the types of omega-3 most important to our health.

If you eat 2–3 servings of fatty fish per week and limit your omega-6 consumption, then you're doing great! If you don't eat enough fish, then a fish oil supplement is a good addition to your diet, and should help keep inflammation in check. Look for a supplement that gives you about 300 mg of combined EPA and DHA per capsule, and aim for 2–4 capsules per day during times when you're not eating enough fatty fish. You don't have to calculate it perfectly.

Flax, chia, hemp, and other plant-based omega-3s – While these foods do have omega-3s in them, they are a form that humans cannot effectively use. A plant-based omega-3 is known as ALA, or alpha-linolenic acid, which must be converted to EPA and DHA by the body, but humans don't do it well. In the case of fish, they've done the work (and conversion) for us!

If you can't eat fish, try krill oil. If you don't eat animal products, look for algae oil instead. If that's not an option, it's even more important to minimize sources of omega-6s. Remember, the two omegas use the same enzymatic pathway for conversion, so the more omega 6s you're processing, the less room your body has to convert ALA to EPA and DHA. Go ahead and take an ALA supplement, but be sure to minimize omega-6s! Seriously.

Omega-3, -6, -9 Supplements – Omega-6s are ubiquitous in our diets, so don't take more of them! Omega-9s are easily produced in the body, and we hardly need any to begin with. Omega-3s sound like a good add, but not when more 6s come along for the ride. Stick with fish, fish oil, krill oil, algae oil. Done.

Grassfed beef and omega-3 eggs – While these foods are often touted as being rich in omega-3s fats, they are not. The truth is they are only higher than *conventionally* raised beef and eggs, but still very low.

Your tasks for this chapter:

1. Consider the fats that you're eating and cooking with. Use your journal to write down several days' worth of food and investigate the fats that are in your meals. See where you can make better choices.

2. Eating out? Consider what goes into the food, but more importantly consider what it's cooked in. If it's deep-fried, you can be pretty sure that it's cooked in low-quality, seed-based oils!

3. Take this knowledge into your kitchen. Cook more and take control of your health (and your pocketbook). When choosing a healthy fat or oil for cooking, there are two basic considerations: taste and smoke point. For most people, olive oil, butter, and a little bacon fat are convenient, tasty choices to have around the house. You can find a table of common oil smoke points in the resources section at eatmovelive52.com.

4. Become a label detective. You'll likely notice that most of the mass-market foods – snacks, treats, and desserts – tend to be

made with lesser quality fats that should be minimized, if not totally avoided. So avoid them!

5. Add one healthy fat to your diet this week. (If you like, add two or three!)

Where to next?

1. Don't Have a Cow, Man! (p.86)
2. Sharpen Your Vision (p.316)

12

Don't Have a Cow, Man!

by Roland

How to get more protein without having to eat the whole farm

In the last few decades, dietary fat went from being the villain that causes heart disease and premature death to the savior that gives us energy and helps balance out our hormones. We went from low-fat to moderate-fat diets, with the new guidelines in 2015 even saying we can add eggs back. Whew!

Carbs were the superhero of the 80s, but in the 90s, people were slashing carbs out of their diets like they were toxic. Insulin became a dirty word.

Today it seems like protein is the only macronutrient that hasn't been attacked then defended, eliminated, then added back, hated, then loved. Through thick and thin, through lean and fat, sweet and salty, protein has always found its place at our table.

Yet, most of us still don't get enough.

Enter the average woman

In my nutrition practice, I rarely see men who undereat protein. A guy, even when completely oblivious of his nutrition needs, is more likely to choose a couple of Egg McMuffins and a slice of bacon for breakfast, a pastrami sandwich for lunch, and get extra meatballs with dinner. Men who have read more about fitness might opt for a shake after their workout, choose extra chicken breast to top their salad, and snack on string cheese and nuts. Because men tend to weigh more, and as a result carry more muscle and have bigger appetites, they naturally tend to get more protein even when they don't think about it. The average woman, however, has spent much of her life worried about her weight, avoids eating foods with more fat or calories, and thus is less likely to get enough nutrients and, specifically, protein.

Let's look at a typical client's meal log. Christine is 40 years old, has 15 lbs of weight she wants to get rid of, and exercises 5 hours a week total. She also walks 5 miles a day. Look at an average day's food:

Breakfast

1 slice whole grain toast with honey

1 egg

Total protein: 10 g

Lunch

Kale and quinoa salad with edamame and sesame seeds

Total protein: 12 g

Snack

1 oz almonds

Total protein: 6 g

Dinner

Spaghetti squash with Bolognese sauce

Arugula salad

Total protein: 12 g

Protein for the day: 40 g

Given that Christine's target bodyweight is 140 lbs, 40 grams is very, very low.

After we made some simple changes to her diet, Christine not only started losing weight faster, but she also noticed more energy and less hunger between meals. Her story is very common.

Maybe you know you need protein, but you are afraid of animal protein

The media hasn't helped. Not a week goes by that a reader doesn't email me a link to the media's latest attempt at a red meat takedown. Meat, red meat, processed meat, and animal protein, in general, are often thought to be unhealthy. Most of this is based on myths and misinformation. Some of the myths you may see floating around:

- Meat causes high cholesterol
- More protein causes constipation
- You can't digest more than 30 grams of protein at once
- Too much protein is harmful to the kidneys
- Too much protein leads to low bone density or osteoporosis
- And finally, you only NEED X amount of protein anyway

On the contrary...

Protein makes up about 20% of your body's total mass. Its building blocks are called amino acids. Amino acids are what form the structure of your muscles, your cells, enzymes, transport and immune system proteins, hormones, or serve as energy for the cells. The body is constantly using them to rebuild and restore, and so it's our job to be good stewards and supply plenty of protein with our food.

It's remarkable how many aspects of our lives improve with adequate protein intake – from all-day energy, to athletic performance, to mental and hormonal health.

If you exercise frequently or have an active life with lots of natural movement, or you are dieting, your needs for protein increase dramatically. Think back to my client – she was eating less than half of what she needed and as soon as we increased her intake, dramatic change started happening, but why?

The many benefits of protein

Protein helps you burn more calories – Your body uses more calories to digest protein than fats and carbs. Veteran calorie counters might say, "But protein is four calories per gram, just like carbohydrate." That's true in a lab, but in the body, which is not as efficient as a lab, we get to burn about 20–30% more calories digesting protein! Higher protein meals increase the metabolic rate for hours after eating, and when you combine higher protein with resistance training, the effect is amplified further.

Protein aids in building and retaining muscle – Protein is the building block of muscle tissue. Even people who don't want big muscles need strong and healthy muscles to be mobile today and independent later in life.

Protein increases bone density – The myth that too much protein makes bones weak is just that, a myth. Higher protein diets have actually been shown to produce more bone mass and fewer fractures.

Protein helps exercise recovery – Protein is required to rebuild and recover after exercise. Lower protein intakes leave you sore longer and less likely to recover in time for your next workout.

Protein is satiating and more filling than other foods – I saved the best for last. At least the best if you're dieting and tired of being hungry. Protein is one of the most filling, satisfying, and satiating things you can eat. It makes you full faster and keeps you less hungry between meals.

How much protein is enough protein?

There's no magic number. Our good friend, nutritionist Alan Aragon says that 0.5 grams to 1 gram per pound of target bodyweight (what you actually want to weigh) is a good range for most active people (and you know you should be active, right?). Some athletes and bodybuilders tend to go far higher, but research shows that it's probably not necessary even for them, much less for us.

For someone with a 175-pound weight goal, that's anywhere from 88 grams of protein (easy) all the way up to 175 grams (you'll probably have to focus).

	For .5 g per pound	Grams of protein	For 1 g per pound	Grams of protein
Breakfast	2 eggs, 3 strips of bacon	21 g	3 eggs, 4 strips of bacon	30 g
Lunch	chicken salad with 4oz chicken	36 g	chicken salad with 6oz chicken	52 g
Dinner	4oz steak	24 g	8oz steak	48 g
Snack	Greek yogurt, carrots	10 g	Greek yogurt, carrots	20 g
Snack	not necessary	0 g	protein shake	25 g
Total		**91 grams**		**175 grams**

Let's see what that looks like.

Half to 1 gram per pound of bodyweight is quite a big range, but that's a good thing. You don't have to feel like a failure if you don't max out your protein every day...but high fives if you do.

EAT WELL, MOVE WELL, LIVE WELL

Some challenges with eating enough protein

More protein can get expensive – That can be especially true if you try to get your extra protein from fancy cuts of steak or eating at trendy farm-to-table restaurants.

Yes, steak is a great way to get more protein, but the protein in steak isn't better than the protein in other meats. If you love beef, that's fine, but save the steaks for a splurge and choose less expensive cuts for your daily meals. Similarly, the fact that a chicken breast is low in fat doesn't make it a healthier source of protein. The most expensive cut of chicken can also tank your grocery budget while doing nothing for your goals. Dark-meat chicken, canned tuna, pork roasts, protein powders, and nutritionally rich eggs are great and inexpensive sources of protein.

I'm getting too full – For most of our readers, this is a great problem to have. Most want to eat less and feel satisfied, and eating more protein can be a great way to do it. Of course, if you're full before you finish your protein, then you're not accomplishing your goal. The idea isn't just to eat less overall, but to eat more protein and reap the benefits.

Make a swap – Instead of merely eating more protein, try to swap that protein in instead of something else. For most of us, carbs are the best swap. Trade out your bread, rice, fries, sodas, and chips for extra servings of protein.

Protein first – Try eating your protein first. Since it takes a while for your stomach and your brain to agree on whether you're full, use it to your advantage, saving optional foods for last.

Breakfast is tough – Eggs and breakfast meats tend to be higher in fat (even if it's healthy fat), so eating more isn't always best. Instead of worrying about getting enough protein at each meal, distribute your protein over the day. You can eat less protein at one meal and eat more at another. Your body doesn't really care how your protein is distributed, so go lighter at breakfast and make up for it later. You can also try swapping out typical breakfast protein choices like sausage and bacon for higher protein foods like Greek yogurt, ham, and leftover lean meats from last night's dinner.

Lunches are easy, even if not always exciting – You have options, from soups and stews and leftovers from home to bunless burgers, omelets at that place with the "Breakfast served all day" sign, and ordering meat and veggies a la carte at your favorite restaurant.

I'm not used to eating enough protein – This is legit. Protein is pretty filling when you're eating it, and keeps you full longer. This is a blessing and a curse for those of us who want to eat more of it, but once you get your portions up, the curse will be broken! Build up your portions over time if necessary, and remember to eat your protein first.

High-protein snacks – If you eat more satisfying meals, you won't need the snacks as much. Also remember that protein doesn't have to be distributed equally across every meal and snack. Still, jerky, cottage cheese, and Greek yogurt are higher protein snack options. Cheese and nuts are lower in protein, but can be very satisfying and convenient for the healthy snacker.

Great protein sources

I'm going to list foods that are healthy and easy to fit into your diet, but remember, "best" is relative and depends on your likes and preferences.

Animal sources of protein are easy. Chicken and turkey breast have long been go-to protein sources for the dieter because they are inexpensive, lean, and low in calories, but pork tenderloin and many types of fish fall into these categories, too. You can always check out the deli section for cold cuts. Four to 6 ounces of sliced sandwich meat makes a great protein-rich snack.

Dairy is another great option, with whey protein powder leading the charge when it comes to versatility and low cost. Greek yogurt and cottage cheese are also great dairy options.

If you can't handle dairy, look for egg, beef, pea, rice, and hemp protein powders at your natural food store.

Don't forget that foods like eggs, steak, fatty fish, shellfish, dark-meat poultry, bacon, sausage, and cheese, yogurt, kefir, and other dairy products are rich in protein, too, but also tend to have more fat or carbohydrates. These protein sources are still healthy ones, and contain nutrition beyond the protein itself, so don't be afraid to include them in your diet.

Vegetarians can sometimes find it hard to get enough protein from plants alone, so don't be afraid to supplement with powders, beans, lentils, and other legumes. The healthfulness of soybeans, tofu, and tempeh are often debated in nutrition circles, but they can be part of a balanced vegetarian diet. The healthiest soy foods are from fermented soy, like tempeh.

If you prefer to get your protein from plant sources, be sure to use a food log to make sure you are taking in enough protein.

To compare the protein quality of different foods you can look up the PDCAAS (Protein Digestibility Corrected Amino Acid Score) online.

Your tasks for this chapter:

1. Use your journal to write down several days' worth of food. Online calculators or smartphone apps can help you estimate whether you are undereating.

2. Gently bump up your protein intake. If you are really off the mark, adding 20 grams or so every couple of weeks is great. The more active you are, the more you will need.

3. Some benefits of more protein can be almost immediately obvious (less hunger), while others take time to show (weight loss, extra muscle, and gorgeous hair). Still others require you to have faith. You might not notice extra bone density for a couple of years, for instance. In your logs, notes, or journal, keep an eye on the things that change over the next few weeks, and have confidence that the longer term benefits *will* come. When you look back at yourself after a year or more of getting more protein, know that under the skin, you're the healthier and stronger person you want to be.

Where to next?

1. What the Tooth? (p.325)
2. Intermittent Fasting (p.278)

Drink Coffee. Not Too Much. Mostly Black.

by Roland

13

One of the world's most studied drinks might also be one of the healthiest

We have a love-hate relationship with coffee. We love coffee, and we hate it when we are told we can't drink it.

Years ago, coffee was labeled "bad," and the studies of the day seemed to show that coffee drinking came with all sorts of terrible consequences. Lucky for us, scientists and researchers soon realized that people who tended to drink coffee also were more likely to smoke, eat poorly, and exercise less. When they plugged this new info into their studies, they were able to filter things better, and see that the coffee wasn't the problem after all.

These days, we are seeing studies showing the positives that come from drinking coffee, but you'd never know it from talking to friends, family, and clients, most of whom still claim to be "trying to cut back."

Coffee is the elixir of the gods

The things we love tend to get studied. Chocolate, wine, and coffee are three of the most studied vices, and when a new study gets published, the media loves to report on it. This is one area where good news in the media might actually beat out the bad!

Coffee is a complex little bean, containing many special compounds and anti-oxidants, and studies keep coming out positive when it comes to its benefits. Coffee consumption has been linked to lower risks of prostate, breast, and liver cancers, increased cognitive and emotional benefits, such as reduced incidence of Parkinson's disease and depression, plus various metabolic benefits like a lowered risk of type 2 diabetes and metabolic syndrome.

Coffee is one of the most potent sources of anti-oxidants in the human diet, and "superfoods" such as kale, goji berries, and açaí pale in comparison. Overall, coffee seems to have positive effects on inflammation and oxidative damage to DNA, so it's no surprise that the health benefits of coffee are so wide ranging. More coffee isn't necessarily better, but there seem to be few reasons not to drink it, and plenty of reasons to.

While I do think coffee can be a valuable part of a healthy diet and lifestyle, I would be remiss if I didn't also let you know about a few of the negatives.

Good coffee, bad coffee

As much as I hate to say it, there is some evidence against coffee, even if the evidence *for* consuming it is far greater.

- In some people, *unfiltered* coffee can raise cholesterol, especially in those people with a genetic disposition to high cholesterol. Researchers don't know exactly why paper filters are better in this case, but paper filters are much finer than other filters and are also able to absorb oils and compounds that slide right by metal, glass, and plastic. If you have cholesterol concerns, stick to coffee brewed with paper filters, and minimize your espresso drinks, French press coffees, and coffee made with reusable filters.

- Coffee can contain mycotoxins (a toxic substance produced by mold or fungus), but before you ditch your morning joe, consider that many other things contain them, too. Corn, nuts, nut butters, and anything made with grains and seeds can contain mycotoxins. Chocolate and dried fruits can, too. Truth be told, many of these foods contain a lot more mycotoxin than coffee does – in fact most of the foods that we eat contain "toxins" in small amounts, and always have. Coffee producers have known how to best combat the mycotoxin problem for generations. Proper drying, storage, and roasting reduces the molds that produce these toxins, which is a great reason to seek out properly grown and roasted beans. They are not only lower in toxins, but taste better, too.

- While coffee is gluten free, some very gluten-sensitive people find that coffee can cause a cross-reaction. It's rare, but some people with Celiac disease report that coffee causes similar problems to eating foods that contain gluten. Whether it's from gluten/coffee cross-contamination at the plant or a true cross-reaction could be dependent on the sensitivity of the individual. If you've gone gluten free and still flare up, it might be time to consider your coffee consumption. Try 30–60 days coffee free and see how you feel at the end. If you choose to reintroduce it, take it slowly.

- Coffee is not making you fat, but what *you* call coffee might be. Many of my clients and readers think coffee is fattening, but when I ask them what coffee they drink (lattes, mochas, frappuccinos), there's usually very little coffee in there. Calling these drinks coffee is like calling a beer a bottle of water or a bowl of sugar a beet salad.

- Caffeine is a diuretic, yes, but only when you're new to caffeine. Over time, your body adapts, and if you consistently drink about the same amount of coffee, it no longer has a diuretic effect, so don't worry.

- Caffeine is addictive. Yes, however, a moderate amount of coffee is unlikely to be a problem, especially when you look at all the benefits that come with coffee. If you feel the addiction, take a 30-day break and then reintroduce coffee in moderation.

Butter in your coffee?

Yes, butter is healthy, but that doesn't mean you should add it to everything. And to the claims that "'butter coffee'" can improve health? Probably only if it helps you lose weight or you were eating a diet that was too low-fat, which is unlikely. Doctors Spencer and Kasey Nadolsky have found that some of their healthiest patients were experiencing sky high cholesterol numbers after adding butter coffee to their otherwise healthy diets. A return to a diet of more balanced fats and foods resulted in a return to healthy cholesterol levels.

The doctors suggest that while whole food sources of saturated fat are not a problem in most people, "the highly concentrated saturated fat bomb" that comes with 400–600 calories of butter, coconut oil, or MCT oil coffees is likely the culprit that sends blood markers dangerously high.

Does it taste good?

Yes and no, but that can be said for any coffee drink. Luckily coffee and butter are not a magical combination, so there's no need to add it to your diet for health or fat loss. If you love the taste, keep in mind that it's primarily the butter that has the taste. MCT oil has very little taste, so you can just skip it, but be sure to truly skip it, and not just replace it with more butter.

If you want to have butter coffee because you enjoy it, enjoy it in moderation, in small amounts, with a meal, and *in place* of other added fats, not in addition.

Good coffee gone bad

When I tell you coffee is good for you, I mean coffee at its most basic level: coffee from properly grown, processed, and roasted beans, brewed well, and not adulterated with ingredients that are not healthy. In a nutshell, coffee is healthy, but what you do to your coffee might not be.

Flavored coffee – That raspberry crème or vanilla hazelnut ground coffee – any flavored coffee – is likely made with low-quality beans, produced with chemical processes, and flavored with artificial flavors. There's probably nothing raspberry or hazelnut about the added flavors, and because the quality is in question, so is the healthfulness of the coffee. If you must have flavored coffee, add your own flavoring during brewing or in your cup, using spices or natural flavorings and extracts.

Cheap coffee – It's cheap for a reason, because it's often made with cheaper, low-quality Robusto beans, which are bitter and have much more caffeine. If better Arabica beans are used to make the good-tasting coffees that you're used to, they might keep costs low by growing them using a lot of pesticides, and rushing them through processing, increasing the risk of mycotoxins. Cheap coffee is often over-roasted to mask the inferior flavor, but you end up with a bitter taste nonetheless.

Coffee treats – There's nothing wrong with a treat now and then, but if your daily coffee is a mocha, blended coffee drink, or high-calorie vanilla crème brûlée latte, you're no longer drinking coffee, you're having dessert. At this point, all the sugar and additives likely cancel out any of the health benefits of what little coffee you're actually getting, not to mention the hundreds of extra calories you're getting from sugar.

Non-dairy creamers – Most of these actually DO still contain dairy in the form of processed casein from milk and are not a good substitute for milk or cream. Most creamers are merely sugary liquids made from cheap soybean oil, sweeteners, and artificial flavorings. They have a lot of calories and make your otherwise healthy drink unhealthy. If you're lactose intolerant or vegan, choose coconut-, almond-, rice-, or even soymilk-based, low-sugar milks or creamers – not artificially flavored sweet treats.

Your tasks for this chapter:

Michael Pollan famously said, "Eat food. Not too much. Mostly plants," and I believe with a slight adjustment it makes a great directive for coffee.

1. Drink coffee

Search out and buy coffee that's grown well, roasted with care, decaffeinated safely if decaffeinated, and not laced with nasty chemicals and artificial flavorings. Local roasters are popping up everywhere, and these roasters take their coffee seriously. Ask them, and they will share the wheres, hows, and whys of their great-tasting beans.

If you can't find great beans locally, check out eatmovelive52.com for some online sources.

2. Not too much

Most studies show that just one cup of coffee has positive effects, but several studies also showed that even six cups were not a problem for health. In our house, we drink a lot of good decaf, since we don't want to go overboard on the caffeine.

Addicted? Are you letting coffee run your life? Do you need coffee just to wake up? Do you need it just to stay awake? Then it might be time to take a break! I generally suggest a 30–60-day break from all caffeine if you're addicted to coffee.

3. Mostly black

This week, try to find a bean and brew style that lets you enjoy coffee black.

It took me a while to enjoy black coffee, but after finding a bean that I enjoyed, black coffee became enjoyable, too. I still enjoy a latte every few weeks, and I love a little half-and-half some mornings. Galina limits dairy, but enjoys coconut milk and some of the new coconut milk creamers in her coffee.

There's nothing wrong with adding milk, cream, or half-and-half to your coffee, but be aware of the added calories. The same goes for sugar.

If your coffee only tastes good with sweet junk in it, seek out and buy better coffee. If you really love it sweet, try to cut back over time, and try less harmful and less caloric sweeteners.

If you really love flavored coffee, add flavor yourself, during or after brewing. Most people have cinnamon, nutmeg, and baking extracts at home, which are far healthier than the artificial flavorings used in most flavored coffees.

Where to next?

1. Take the Soda Challenge (p.38)
2. Hanging (p.197)

Something Fishy This Way Comes

by Roland

14

A look at the world's most notorious superfood

Has there ever been a more confusing health food than fish? The news headlines and health recommendations are all over the place. Eat your fish; watch the mercury; get your omega-3s; wild caught is best; is farmed fish more sustainable; what are PCBs, anyway?

Even with the confusing health points, pro and con, we have the issues of the taste, the smell, and the cooking of the fish. People are rightfully confused, and when people get confused, they give up.

Fish is a great source of healthy protein, and cold-water, fatty fish are some of the best sources of essential omega-3s you can find. Protein builds muscle, helps your bone density, aids in exercise recovery, and when it comes to weight loss, protein is more satiating than carbohydrate or fat. Omega-3s are a fat that keeps our brains and bodies healthy. They reduce inflammation, keeping us pain free. They lessen the chances of diseases of age and of the mind affecting us before our time.

But fish are contaminated

True, but so is everything else!

We live in a world where virtually every food we eat is contaminated by *something* toxic. Leafy greens, for instance, are the food most likely to make you sick, but we don't avoid eating them. We all know that eating leafy greens is important, so we're smart about it. We choose our greens wisely, and wash them well.

Eating fish is as important as eating leafy greens, and making smart choices about fish isn't as hard as we think.

What are the big contamination concerns when it comes to fish?

Mercury

Yes, fish has mercury, but you can't look at mercury in fish in isolation. Mercury doesn't tell the whole story. Selenium plays a big part, too. It's a bit complicated, but in the end, you're more likely to have mercury issues from fish if you're deficient in selenium. Luckily, many fish also come loaded with selenium!

As you can see in the graph, only the shark (on the far right) is an issue. Most of us don't eat much shark, and there's really no reason to start with so many healthier fish to choose from.

We also recommend that you get selenium from other foods. For instance, just 2–3 Brazil nuts per week can provide enough selenium for most people's needs!

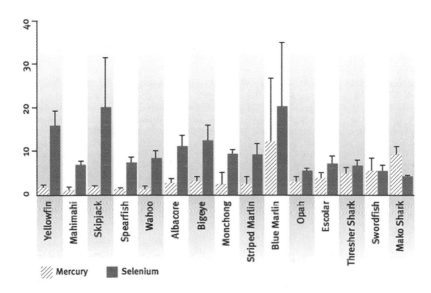

This chart is created by the Western Pacific Regional Fishery Management Council. For the detailed chart in entirety, please visit eatmovelive52.com.

PCBs and dioxins

While it's true that fish contain toxins like PCBs and dioxins, foods such as dairy, vegetables, beef, pork, and chicken all contain several times more. Even then, the biggest concern is a perceived increased risk of cancer, but the reduction in heart disease (CHD) risk that comes from eating fish far outweighs the risk of cancer.

"Per 100 000 individuals, consumption of farmed vs wild salmon would result in 24 vs 8 excess cancer deaths, respectively, while consumption of either farmed or wild salmon would result in 7125 fewer CHD deaths" (Fish Intake, Contaminants, and Human Health, Evaluating the Risks and the Benefits, *JAMA*. 2006;296[15]).

Radiation

While it's true that the Japanese nuclear meltdown has contaminated fish in the Pacific Ocean, the actual contamination levels of the fish are very low.

Scientists studied fish that had migrated from Japan to San Diego and found that they did contain trace amounts of radiation from Japan, but that the levels of radiation from the incident were thirty times lower than the naturally occurring radiation in the fish.

All foods on Earth naturally contain radiation, and fish actually has a lot less than that banana you recently ate (i.e., not much).

Better safe than sorry?

Yes! And when it comes to fish, the safest thing seems to be to actually eat it.

While a few studies using high-mercury, low-selenium fish (often whale, which is not even a fish) show some negatives, many other studies show that mothers who eat high levels of seafood have healthier children, with better motor development and higher IQs.

In fact, a study of 14,000 mother-child pairs found that the children of mothers who had eaten less than 12 ounces of fish per week had more significant impairments of communication skills when young, and that lower verbal IQs and communications skills continued on to adolescence.

While some reports of contamination have suggested an increased risk of some diseases, the actual increased risk was insignificant compared to the increased life expectancy from *adding* more fish to your diet. Not to mention the cognitive benefits and lowered risk of diseases like dementia and Alzheimer's that come from a diet rich in the omega-3s found in fish.

Yes, eating more fish was better and eating less fish was worse. Now let's take a look at some of the best fish choices out there.

Choosing the best fish for omega-3s

Fatty, cold-water fish are the best sources of omega-3s, so choose salmon, mackerel, herring, sardines, and anchovies. Aim for at least 2–3 servings per week.

Farmed salmon is still healthy, but not as healthy as wild salmon. Farmed fish are fed fish meal, which is cheap calories, not healthy food. More importantly, farmed fish are also overcrowded and fed antibiotics to keep them healthy. As a result, their fat makeup is not as good, their toxin levels are higher, and the farms themselves are environmentally devastating. While farmed fish might seem to be a good compromise, they really aren't.

Tuna is often called a good source of omega-3s, and while its fats are good, tuna simply isn't very fatty. It's healthy and a great source of protein, but if you want your omega-3s, be sure to eat fatty fish, too.

What if I just can't do fish?

If you can't or won't eat enough fatty fish (2–3 servings per week), then a quality fish oil, krill oil, or algae oil supplement is important.

Fish oil – I prefer capsules because of the convenience. Kirkland/Costco is a good source of fish oil capsules at a reasonable cost. Because of the high turnover, their fish oil tends to be fresh, and Consumer Reports gave it high ratings when analyzed. If you prefer liquid fish oil, look for one that's flavored with lemon or another flavoring to cover up the fish taste.

Krill oil – Krill oil is more costly, but a good solution for people who are allergic to fish. Fish get a lot of their omega-3s from krill. I can't think of a higher endorsement!

Algae oil – Algae oil is where krill get *their* omega-3s. Talk about going to the source.

Even if you do eat fish, it can't hurt to have a supplement in the fridge, for those weeks when you mean to eat fish, but never get around to it.

Choosing the best fish for protein

Tuna has long been a favorite of bodybuilders due to its high protein content, good taste, canned or packaged convenience, and because of its relatively low price. It's also easy to have on hand, since it lasts for years in the can.

Fresh or frozen, fish like mahimahi, halibut, sea bass, sole, and tilapia are all great sources of protein because they have so little fat. Because the fats in fish are so healthy, I hate to tell you to look for low-fat fish, but the reality is that if you're dieting and trying to get more protein, lower fat fish are a good choice.

Just be sure to still eat your fatty fish in addition to eating fish for protein. There's no substitute in your diet for omega-3s, so find a lesser fat, like cheap salad dressings, soybean or corn oil, to skip, and make room for fatty fish.

Choosing the best fish for the environment

Farmed fish vs. wild-caught fish is a contentious issue. On one hand, wild-caught fish are healthier, both themselves and for us to eat, but catching them is dangerously reducing some species of fish. On the other hand, farm-raised fish require heavy doses of antibiotics, are overcrowded, and pollute the surrounding areas with their waste.

Solutions on both sides are being sought, but in the meantime I choose to eat fish that are the most sustainable, like wild-caught salmon and mackerel, sardines, anchovies, and herring. Thankfully, these are also some of the best sources of omega-3 fats.

One great source of information on the sustainability of fish is the Monterey Bay Aquarium's Seafood Watch at www.seafoodwatch.org. In addition to charts for your local area, they have on online, interactive sushi and seafood selection guide, downloadable guides and recommendations, and even a smartphone app!

Best fish for people who don't like fish

Least fishy fish – tilapia, snapper, sole, canned tuna, mahimahi

Most like meat – tuna steaks, ahi steaks, halibut, swordfish

Most of the least fishy fish are also low in fat, fish oil, and omega-3s, so be sure to have a good fish oil supplement, as well.

Still have fears?

Have some selenium – Brazil nuts are the winner when it comes to selenium, and 2–3 Brazil nuts per week is more than enough to serve as your selenium safety net and help protect you from mercury. Other good sources are beef, pork, and chicken, but you only need to eat an ounce of Brazil nuts to get the same amount of selenium as you'd find in five steaks.

Also note that mercury is stored in the meat of the fish, not the fat, so…

Choose small and fatty fish – Smaller, fattier fish tend to be lower on the food chain, and have eaten fewer other fish and hence fewer contaminants. Sardines, herring, and anchovies are pretty small, and in the grand scheme of things, even a salmon is small. When it comes to tuna, choose chunk light tuna, which comes from the smaller, younger tuna. Chunk white is from bigger tuna, and solid white from bigger tuna still.

Again, the less fatty fish you eat, the more you have to rely on fish oil for omega-3s.

But aren't grassfed beef, omega-3 eggs, and flaxseeds good sources of omega-3s?

I'm afraid not.

There are great reasons to choose grassfed beef over conventional beef, but omega-3s aren't one of them. While grassfed beef does contain several times the amount of omega-3s that feedlot beef contains, it's still a tiny amount, and not a significant source of 3s. (Check out our Good Fat, Bad Fat chapter for more on omegas.)

Your tasks for this chapter:

1. Choose 1 or 2 types of fish that you'd like to try. If you like fish but you've been afraid to eat it, I hope you've been convinced that it's not only safe to eat fish, but safer to eat it than to not eat it. You can find preparation instructions and recipes in the resources section at eatmovelive52.com

2. If you already like the taste of fish, or once you're more accustomed to it, add more fatty fish to your diet.

Where to next?

1. Walking Like Nature Intended (p.154)
2. Ferment Your Food (p.124)

15 Tame Your Sugar Monster by Galina

Face down your sugar addiction, learn to control it, and teach it to behave

Ten years ago, my gym started carrying a performance-enhancing sweet beverage. I was an overall sensible eater, watched my calories and macronutrients, and made sure I didn't eat a lot of processed food, but I didn't understand the addictive nature of sweet things. The first time I tasted Cherry Fever, it was a free sample. It tasted a bit like chemicals and left a tart cherry, sweet aftertaste. I didn't particularly like it even after finishing the whole bottle. When I tried another free sample, Wild Orange flavor, I didn't particularly like that either.

By the end of the week, I had tried all flavors and was wildly in love with them. I would wake up planning my meals around having one or two of these drinks while I was at the gym. By the end of a month, I was considering getting cases of them to take home.

I was also starting to buy more flavored yogurts, and was regularly adding honey to my oatmeal. At night, chocolate was talking to me from the cupboard. Lindt truffles were calling my name at grocery store checkout lines.

At the time I was leading a corporate wellness program at a large soft drink and juice company. One day I shared with their marketing manager how addicted I had become to that sports drink. She explained that they have a whole research team that has determined the number of times you need to be exposed to a free sample in order to start liking it and then buying it.

And then it hit me: I had gotten myself accustomed to the sweet taste. Once addicted my body had started to expect a fix every day and sometimes once every few hours. The drink's sweetness and flavor had opened a door and invited other sweet treats into my life.

What's the deal with sugar?

Throughout millions of years of evolution, our species has become conditioned to seek out the sweet taste. Mother's milk, the very substance on which life grows, is mostly sweet. There isn't just a physiological, but also an emotional connection to the sweet taste in terms of comfort and safety. Once weaned off mother's milk, to find similar taste we had to look for foods that were sweet; however, in nature, forest fruits, dates, and honey are few and far between. Think of gathering substantial quantities of wild strawberries, dates, figs, or honey (protected by bees) – the amounts available to us would have been relatively small, seasonal, and probably cost a ton of energy to obtain. Fruit, as we know it today, available at the farmer's market, is the product of careful selection, weeding out bitter and sour tastes, and replacing it with sweet taste. Our instinctive preference for sweet foods developed in an environment where those foods were rare, yet today that instinct is still with us in an environment that abounds in sweets.

How sugar drives behavior

Sugar drives behavior in two ways – on one hand we have the addictive properties of the "feel good" brain chemicals that get released when we consume sweet foods and drinks. On the other hand, sugar has a direct biological effect on our blood sugar regulation, hunger and satiety signals, as well as energy levels. Eating foods that are high in sugar provides an initial surge in blood sugar and energy. However, to cope with it the pancreas has to release more insulin than it would for a meal that had a more moderate amount of sugar, clearing it as quickly as possible from the bloodstream. As blood sugar and energy levels drop, we are driven to eat again so that we feel better, whether we actually need the calories or not.

You may have noticed this yourself, eating a peanut butter and jelly sandwich for breakfast, then grabbing a piece of chocolate from someone's desk, then going for a cookie right before lunch. You have a physical sensation of hunger and low energy even though you have consumed food recently and surely don't need the calories. Some people (like me and about 80% of my clients) are particularly sensitive – even a small amount of sugar eaten on an empty stomach can create a cascading effect and make energy unstable for the whole day.

Sugary foods sabotage our health in three ways: They may create an addictive desire for more food, when there is no deficit, thus creating a pattern of overconsumption. Second, they may create fluctuations in blood sugar, which leads to unstable energy and the

Stephan Guyenet of Whole Health Source was the researcher who allowed us to really get a good grip on how food choices shape behavior, by explaining food palatability and food reward. Palatability, also known as hedonic value, has to do with how much enjoyment we get from a food. For example, a high-quality steak is palatable to a lot of people, and you may find yourself craving it. Yet, you can get full and have enough steak, without wanting to have it over and over and over again soon. However, if certain brain chemicals that have to do with repeat behavior get triggered, then we talk about food reward – a quality that makes us motivated to seek those foods out and want them a lot. Chocolate is both palatable and rewarding to a lot of people, while steak may be palatable, yet not specifically rewarding. Imagine finishing a dinner at a restaurant, after eating a salad and a main dish. You are satisfied and full. The waitress comes by and offers you a free bowl of rice. Would you say yes? What if it wasn't rice, but a molten chocolate brownie? What might you say to that, full or not?

desire to eat sooner than we need. And third, industrial or manufactured foods high in sugar provide very little nutrition in terms of usable vitamins, minerals, enzymes, or phytonutrients. You may have heard the term "empty calories" referring to processed and high-sugar foods – they provide energy that is not accompanied by the nutrients that the body actually needs. This can create further behavior changes, such as overeating, driving the overconsumption of more of those empty calories. The body is starving for nutrients, yet is overfed calories.

In the name of sugar

Sugar has many names, from the plain old white sugar on Grandma's table to any of the following: agave nectar, brown rice syrup, high-fructose corn syrup, corn syrup, molasses, honey, cane juice, maple syrup, sucrose, glucose, fructose, dextrose, maltose, lactose, caramel, coconut sugar, fruit juice concentrate, galactose, invert sugar, maltodextrin. It's helpful to know those names so that you have an easier time reading labels and knowing when a food contains sugar. (To really become a good label detective, refer to the chapter Ingredient Espionage.)

What to do next?

Spend some time thinking about your main priorities: Do you want to lose weight, simply eat better, enjoy more energy, manage a health problem or genetic predisposition related to sugar such as diabetes, heart disease, Alzheimer's, or cancer? Or do you just want to base your food decisions on real signals of hunger and not be a puppet of addictive substances?

Clean up your act

To re-establish a healthy relationship with sugar will take some time. We recommend you take two to four weeks off of any added sugars in your drinks, off juice, soft drinks, cookies, pastries, chocolates, doughnuts, and the like.

It's possible that you will miss the sweet taste quite a bit at first. When in need of the sweet taste opt for plenty of berries, such as strawberries, raspberries, blackberries, blueberries, and cherries. Instead of orange juice, have a whole orange; instead of apple pie, bake some apples with cinnamon.

Opt for naturally sweet-tasting teas, such as hibiscus, licorice, rooibos, and chamomile.

Chocolate lovers may find that a cup of hot coconut milk made with natural, unsweetened cocoa powder or cacao nibs on yogurt are great ways to get the natural, rich flavors of chocolate, minus the high sugar content.

During your time of transition, whether you go for two or four weeks, it's crucial to provide your body with excellent nutrition to stabilize your blood sugar and secure stable energy levels.

Make protein, vegetables, and healthy fats the base of each meal. Eggs with breakfast, chicken with lunch, and fish with dinner, alongside rich, colorful salads sprinkled with seeds and nuts are a great way to be full and satisfied and forget about sugar.

Naturally sweet vegetables such as cooked tomatoes, squash, corn, and onions will definitely be your best friends during this time. To kick it up one more notch, add sweet-tasting spices such as vanilla, cinnamon, nutmeg, allspice, and ginger to stews and soups, yogurt, and cooked fruit.

Inviting sugar back into your life

Our relationship with food is so rich and complex. It goes beyond what's good for us, what our culture accepts as normal, or even what we know makes us sick in the wrong amounts. The coffee date over flavored cappuccino with whipped cream, the sundae you share with your sister on every birthday, the warm cookies your mom makes every Christmas, and that cake recipe everyone raves about so much that you make it over and over again – so many of our emotions, memories, and history are tied to food.

The majority of our clients choose to reintroduce some sugary foods into their lives even after they have determined that they have been eating sugar out of addictive behavior, boredom, or to compensate for unstable energy levels.

After several weeks off sweets, most people find that foods they previously considered sweet are now overwhelmingly sweet. Taste receptors have experienced a reset and now food tastes different. If they also learn how to savor food, and take the time to mindfully enjoy it, small amounts are now enough to satisfy a desire, create the atmosphere for a family event, or to bring guaranteed joy at the end of a hard day.

Follow these rules for embracing sugar

Never eat sweets on an empty stomach – Make sure that you have a good base of protein and vegetables waiting in your stomach, so that when sugar enters the scene the speed at which it elevates your blood glucose is nice and smooth, versus creating sharp spikes and drops.

When you do eat them, choose the highest quality sweets – Peanut butter cups are a good example. Our local Starbucks carries organic peanut butter cups covered in dark or white chocolate – the textures and flavors are deep and rich and the pleasure is truly worth it.

Be present with your food – Notice texture, tastes, flavor, the way it melts, the way it goes down your throat. Wait for one bite to fully dissolve and for the taste to dissipate before you go to the next bitc.

Keep track of sugar – Track your grams or calories. In general 25 grams of sugar or a treat between 100 and 200 calories won't create too much havoc if enjoyed a couple of times a week.

Time your sugar intake – The body expends a lot of energy from glucose (the stored form of sugar) during hard exercise, such as steep hiking, sprinting, or resistance training. If you time your sugar intake to follow your hard work, you shouldn't experience such dramatic, negative effects.

Monitor your behaviors – If you notice that you are reaching for sweets mindlessly or that you are eating out of boredom or for emotional reasons, take a step back, journal about it, and maybe take a week off sweets before you invite them into your life again.

Your tasks for this chapter:

1. Look deeply at your motivation to eat sweets. Look even deeper at your motivation to reduce your sugar intake. Journal about it for personal insights.

2. Cut sugary foods out for 2 to 4 weeks.

3. When ready to invite sugar back into your life, make sure that you follow the steps outlined above.

Where to next?

1. Walk More Today (p. 345)
2. Walk More Today is the one of the first four lessons we've hand picked for you. We suggest you give that a try. After the first four, the sky's the limit!

16

Odds and Ends and the Anti-Cancer Soup

by Roland

How eating the parts that most people throw away can be the healthiest way to eat

We have a cancer problem, and the news media think it's all the meat.

Too much meat, too much red meat, too much processed meat, and too much protein. At least, so the headlines say.

Yes, if you read select studies, it can appear that higher protein levels can increase some cancer risks. However, it doesn't appear to be the protein or the meat itself, processed or otherwise, that's to blame. No, it's a lack of a certain amino acid balance in our diet that looks to be the culprit. Specifically, when these amino acids are out of balance our IGF-1 levels go up, which is what can increase the cancer risk.

IGF-1 (insulin-like growth factor 1) is necessary for cell turnover, growth, and healing, but when it gets too high, it's thought to be a contributor to premature aging, shorter lifespans, and to things like cancer growth. Keeping IGF-1 at the right levels certainly has benefits. But what causes IGF-1 levels to rise too high?

Spoiler alert: it's not the meat!

IGF-1 levels can go higher when we eat more protein, but it's not really the protein, the red meat, or the amount that's to blame; it's the *makeup* of the protein. I'm not talking grassfed and pastured vs. corn fed feedlot beef here. I'm not even talking specific animals or even animal vs. vegetable protein. It's the parts of the animal that we eat that's the problem. Actually, it's more like the parts that we *don't* eat.

It turns out that what kicks up our IGF-1 levels are the ratios between some of the amino acids found in protein. These amino acids, the building blocks of protein, occur in varying levels in every protein source we eat. Muscle meats (our favorites, here in the West) are very rich in one of these amino acids, methionine, and very low in glycine and choline. That's not inherently bad...unless all we eat is muscle meat.

In the industrialized, Western world, we tend to eat mostly meat like steaks, roasts, and fillets, all of which, as muscle meats, hike our methionine levels higher and higher. We also tend to skip the odds and ends that have historically played a big role in the human diet. Livers, skin, and bones, among other things, used to be eaten more often than not, either directly, or in the case of bones, after being simmered into a soup. These spare parts tend to contain a large amount of glycine and choline, which would historically balance out our amino acid profile and keep IGF-1 levels low.

Today, as we focus our culinary energy on muscle meat while ignoring the odds and ends, we leave a lot of nutrition on the table, or more likely, in the trash, and that's affecting our health in ways that we are just starting to understand.

The latest from the low-fat legacy

When our cultures went low fat several decades ago, we stopped eating many of the traditional "nose to tail" parts of our food, including the liver, organ meats, and skin. While the loss of healthy fat was kind of a big deal in and of itself, a bigger deal was the loss of the micronutrients and amino acids that are contained within these spare parts.

Glycine-rich foods, whether in the form of poultry skin, a salmon skin roll, pork rinds, or bone broth, play an important role, and shouldn't be considered spare parts, or optional at all. The same goes for liver, even though I know you probably have bad memories from that liver and onions Mom used to make on Sunday. These extras aren't extras; they are healthy, necessary parts of a nutritious diet.

Low protein is not the answer

Some people recommend that we dramatically cut the protein, but protein has too many benefits to pass up. Protein helps in building and maintaining muscle and bone, helps to fill you up faster when you eat, helps you burn extra calories from your food, has been shown to help dieters stay on track with their diets, and increases recovery after a workout. No, eating less protein isn't the best answer, not when there are other, better options.

I'll tell you later...

Spare parts, bits and pieces, livers, organ meats, bones, bone marrow, and skin. Yuck.

At least that's what Americans and many other industrialized cultures say to these foods, today. But take a trip back in time, or around the globe, and you'll find these items on tables and stoves more often than not.

On my last trip to Bulgaria, my friends ordered up platters of unidentifiable meats, thankfully chopped small and well-seasoned with onions, garlic, and plenty of spices. I ate them without question…at first.

When I eventually asked what I was eating, I was told that it was "hard to explain in English," but what they really meant was, "I'll tell you later." I started to get suspicious, but ate up nevertheless. It turned out I was eating tripe, kidneys, intestines, liver, and hearts. There may have been more things on the platters, but I did not try to find a better translator. I'd heard enough already.

I'm an adventurous eater, but even in my case, it sometimes helps to taste first and ask questions later! It also helps to start with the easy stuff and save the rest until you gain more experience.

The healthiest cultures in the world eat gross things

But you don't have to eat gross to eat healthier. There are many glycine- and choline-rich foods that I'm sure you will find delicious, like chicken soup, egg yolks, broth, pâté, liverwurst, and even pork rinds or the skin on chicken! Most people love, or at least like, some of these things, and you just have to eat them more often!

Glycine-rich foods, ranked from easy to make to harder to take

Easy

- Egg yolks. Stop throwing them away, and stop buying egg whites. Done.

- Skin-on poultry, like chicken skin, the skin of ducks, quail, Cornish game hens, turkey, and other birds, pork rinds and chicharrón, and even salmon skin.

- You might notice that most kids naturally eat the skin on chicken until we start telling them to pull it off, so if you have kids, stop telling them! For the rest of us, it's time to start digging in. If you're not used to it, I find drumsticks and wings to be the easiest to start with, and one of the most cost effective meats on the market.

- Pork rinds are a tasty snack, but like many snack foods, they can be ruined by artificial flavors and sketchy ingredients. The best pork rinds and chicharrón are simply cooked in their own fat, so the ingredients will be things like pork, pork skin, pork fat, and salt. Spicy flavored rinds are also available, but they are harder to find free of MSG and artificial flavors and colors.

- Salmon skin is often left behind on plates or pans, but that's the best part, and very healthy.

- Homemade chicken soup or broth, simmered with the skin and bones.

Medium

- Bone broth isn't something we're used to making or eating here in the land of modernity. Most people love broth and stock, but throw in the word "bone" and suddenly we're turned off. There are a million ways to make bone broth, and whole websites dedicated to helping you fine tune the broth, but that's a lot of work and a lot of worry. Keep in mind that Great-Grandma just put it on the stove and simmered it until it was done; she didn't use a digital thermometer, mail order bones, or artesian spring water.

  Yes, you can be a bone broth perfectionist, but the difference between pretty good and perfect is going to be minor. Just make the broth and start cooking with it!

THE DENZELS' BONE BROTH RECIPE

Use 5 lbs of bones – marrow bones are best. Place in a slow cooker and cover with water. Add a tablespoon of apple cider vinegar. Cook on low for at least 12 hours, adding water if necessary. We sometimes cook this broth for 30 hours or so – it positively influences the flavor and mineral content. Once taken off the heat, pour the broth in jars and refrigerate. The fat will freeze on top and will be easy to remove. You can store the broth in the fridge to use for soups, stews, and sautéing. To preserve it longer, you can freeze servings in ice cube trays and store them in zipper bags, and always have small portions on hand to drink or include in recipes. In winter 3–4 cubes with added hot water, lemon juice, and ginger is how Galina starts her day!

Harder

- Organ meats, liver, liverwurst, pâté, braunschweiger. I do not like liver. I grew up eating liverwurst, however, and if it's not clear from the name, it is made of liver. I love it, so I guess I do like liver. That's a dirty trick!

    It's a good thing that there are ways to eat all the miscellaneous, healthiest parts of the animal as part of a food instead of as the food itself. One of the best ways is to take small amounts of the item in question and mix it into foods where it won't be noticed, like chili, sauces, stews, or even meatballs and meatloaf. You can buy sausages made from organ meats online, as well. They just taste like regular ol' sausage.

    While we're on the subject of meatloaf, our friend Angelo Coppola, from HumansAreNotBroken.com, has a recipe for burgers that's a great way to secretly introduce liver to the family, and it can be our little secret. You'll find it in the resource section at eatmovelive52.com.

Your tasks for this chapter:

1. Powerfully increase your nutrition by adding glycine- and choline-rich foods to your diet a couple of times per week. Find opportunities to enjoy glycine rich foods by buying a package of crunchy pork rinds, making a roast chicken and enjoying the skin, or buying salmon fillets with the skin on. Use your journal to plan those foods into your weekly menu and note how they tasted and the recipes you tried!

2. Once you are comfortable with more skin on chicken and fish, go further. Get more choline by eating whole eggs, not egg whites, and shopping in the deli section for liverwurst,

braunschweiger, or pâté. You might have to head to a specialty store for a good variety, but it's worth the effort!

3. Become a bone collector. Chicken bones (and turkey around the holidays) are typically the cheapest and easiest source for bone broth. Start collecting bones and spare parts from the roast chickens you eat, and freeze them in heavy zipper bags until you have enough to fill your pot or slow cooker. Start the conversation with your local butcher, and see about finding a source of beef, lamb, or pork bones. Mail order is also an option for those ordering their meat in bulk.

Where to next?

1. The E-Detox (p.382)
2. Bulletproof Your Low Back (p.223)

17 Ferment Your Foods

by Roland

What our ancestors forgot to throw out

Fermenting has been around since forever. Controlled fermentation – meaning we did it on purpose – has been around for about eight thousand years, if not longer.

Since those ancient times, when that very first molecule of sugar was swarmed over and consumed by yeast and bacteria, fermentation has been happily producing gasses, acids, and alcohol, and we've been happily enjoying the results.

Gut check time!

It might sound gross, but the average human body is home to about 100 trillion bacteria. These bacteria do all sorts of things, from helping you digest your food to boosting your immune system. In some ways, these bacteria *are* your immune system. The various bacteria in your body work together, in balance and harmony, to fight off infections and squash disease before it starts.

Usually, there's a healthy mix of many different bacteria species in and on our bodies at all times. Sometimes our immune systems can get weakened by, for example, lack of sleep, a virus, poor nutrition, overwork, injury, or even stress. One bad strain of bacteria sees an opening and takes over; suddenly we have an infection.

Many of us have suffered through bad infections. The doctor gave us a powerful antibiotic to knock it down, sometimes warning about the possibility of diarrhea or gas, and often recommending that we eat some yogurt as we recover. You might have thought that the yogurt was something to soothe the stomach, and while it might do that, it's actually to repopulate your gut with good bacteria.

While antibiotics do a pretty good job of killing the enemy bacteria that cause our infections, they also tend to kill off a lot of the good bacteria that are on your side. Yogurt, being a fermented, live food, contains colonies of healthy bacteria that are ready to relocate from their short-term home in that little carton, to long-term residence in your belly! Once these healthy colonies of friendly bacteria have been re-established, your antibiotic-induced gas (and worse) goes away. Your gut is healthy again!

Back to the future. Back to the 70s.

People have been making their own yogurt for thousands of years, even before electricity. In the 70s, a health and natural food craze was sweeping the country, and yogurt became the next big thing for people who wanted to feel good and eat right. It was an era filled with wheat germ, granola, nutritional yeast, sprouts, and…yogurt!

Back in the 70s, health food stores and hippies were touting the benefits of eating more natural and traditional foods, and they hit a home run with yogurt. Unfortunately, in the grocery stores of the 70s, most yogurt was flavored with jam and sugar and labeled "fruit on the bottom." Getting high-quality, healthy yogurt was tougher than it is today. Yes, yogurt itself is healthy, but as you've seen in other chapters, even the healthiest foods can be ruined by adding in too many bad guys.

The 70s hippie response to bad yogurt was to make *real* yogurt at home, or on the commune, using traditional methods. Since most of them didn't know how, appliance manufacturers took to the market with electric devices that made seven little cups of yogurt for them while they slept. It did make it easy, and you can still buy similar devices today, but you don't need to. People were making yogurt long before the invention of electricity.

Want to try making your own? Head over to eatmovelive52.com for our tried and true yogurt and Greek yogurt recipes.

Other ferments

Pickles – There are two kinds of pickles; one kind is the type you find on most grocery store shelves, which are pickled (cured, actually) by brining in salt, vinegar, and spices. The other type is pickled via fermentation, and will be found in the refrigerated section, if at all. These are rare in the grocery store, but Bubbies is one brand that makes delicious fermented pickles. Most fermented pickle brands will brag about being fermented somewhere on the label. Fermented pickles are tasty, but very different from salt and vinegar pickles.

Sauerkraut – True sauerkraut is simply fermented cabbage and salt, but most kraut in the supermarket is pickled or brined, not fermented. Pickled kraut is still healthy, like most vegetables are, but it's not rich with the good bacteria of fermented sauerkraut. You can buy fermented sauerkraut at health and natural food stores, but it can be expensive. Fermented kraut is easy and very inexpensive to make, so I encourage you to try.

Kimchi – A spicy Korean vegetable dish, usually made by fermenting combinations of cabbage, daikon radish, garlic, onion, and chili paste. Traditional versions often include some umami-producing fish or shrimp paste and may have been buried in a field until ready to eat!

Kombucha – A fizzy drink of fermented tea that's now so popular it's stocked in traditional grocery store drink coolers. A floating SCOBY (Symbiotic Culture Of Bacteria and Yeast) converts the sugary tea to a tart, bubbly drink over a week or two. If you like store-bought kombucha (GT's is a popular brand), consider making your own at home with a kit purchased online.

Kefir – Many people think kefir is just drinkable yogurt, but it's actually a totally different group of bacteria. Kefir also ferments with yeast and bacteria, and, like kombucha, uses a SCOBY or "mother" as some call it.

I encourage you to eat a variety of fermented foods from the list above, but when it comes to making your own, some fermented foods are complicated, sound sketchy, or both. Some are very simple to make, but when it comes time to taste them...well, we get nervous. Sauerkraut, for instance, is extremely simple, but for some people getting up the nerve to take that first bite is a scary thing. As a culture, we are not used to eating foods that have been left to do their thing on the countertop for a week.

Yogurt does have a few more steps than kraut, but most of us feel confident that we can recognize a safe bite of yogurt when we see it. And for many people, yogurt makes a great starter when it comes to eating and making fermented foods.

Your tasks for this chapter:

1. Do you like yogurt? Venture out of the comfort zone and make it at home.
2. Try one other fermented food – kombucha, if you feel like a refreshing drink, or maybe Bubbies pickles.
3. Check out a book on fermentation from the library, such as *Fermented* by Jill Ciciarelli. In the references section of this book, there are several titles of other books we love.

Where to next?

1. Confessions of a Massage Addict (p.351)
2. Meditate on This (p.340)

The Best Things Come in NO Packages

18

Let fresh food teach you a lesson about real food

My neighbors were gone for two weeks, and it was my job to water their plants and put any packages or newspapers that showed up inside their door. The day after they left, a huge box of produce was delivered by a local Community Supported Agriculture (CSA) service. I took it to my place, knowing it would rot otherwise.

I took each item out and checked it against the included list: purple carrots, golden beets, tomatoes, tiny white potatoes, red leaf lettuce, plums, honeydew melon, a lemon, two peaches, and more. The unidentified leaves I'd seen lurking were an unusual type of spinach and the other stems were actually listed as "greens."

The CSA provided recipes for the more unusual items, and I learned that I could cook these greens with bacon and pepper, and that I could cook other greens (like beet greens) the same way.

Back then, I already considered myself a healthy eater, having lost quite a bit of weight by eating less food and less fat, but my idea of eating my five servings of vegetables and fruit a day was an iceberg salad at lunch, half a can of green beans at dinner, a banana for a snack, and I'd make up the other two tomorrow. Now, faced with a week's worth of free fresh produce, I needed a plan.

Reading the CSA box's recipes, I noticed that most of the recipes were side dishes. I needed something for them to be the side *to*. I made a short grocery list and headed to the store, picking up a pork chop, some boneless chicken thighs, and, of course, some bacon. I also bought a small chuck steak to go with the purple carrots and

NUTRITION   129 tiny potatoes; a take on my mom's beef stew.

The stew was easy because I'd made it before, but what surprised me was how easy it was to take all of this raw produce and turn it into dinners simply by pairing the foods with my favorite meats (most were grilled, out of pure laziness).

In the end, I spent two weeks without cracking open any boxes, yet spent about the same amount of time in my kitchen. By cooking simply, these lazy weeks of cooking weren't really any more work than the weeks before, which were based on the "convenience" of less healthy packaged foods.

What's the problem with packaged food?

Our relationship with packaged foods is complicated, and it's time to face it. Years ago, mac and cheese was a side dish. Today we make a double batch and serve it up as the only food on the table. Where did the main dish go? Where is the chicken? Where are the vegetables? Foods like Hamburger Helper show pictures of a complete meal of pasta and ground beef on the box, with not a vegetable in sight.

These packaged foods are designed to have a long shelf life, be high in profits for the manufacturer, and tasty enough for people to buy them again and again. Food manufacturers tend to use cheap seed oils, inexpensive grains, and lots of artificial and engineered ingredients.

Besides what they put into the packages, it's important to consider what they leave out. Most packaged foods contain very little protein. Protein is expensive and quality protein even more so. Packaged foods also contain few vegetables, relying instead on grain-based carbs for the bulk of the box. Because of the use of inexpensive grains, cheap and unhealthy fats, a small amount of protein, and few vegetables, most of these packages come high in calories and low in nutrition.

Before my spontaneous two weeks without packaged food, my

> ## FOOD PAIRINGS
>
> Some foods go very well together and can become a real food staple at your table and help up your confidence levels in the kitchen. Here are a few of our favorites:
>
> **Pork carnitas** – pair with sauteed peppers and onions, serve with guacamole and lime
>
> **Goat cheese omelet** – pair with tomato, Kalamata olive, and arugula salad
>
> **Meatballs** – pair with tomato sauce over roasted zucchini and eggplant instead of pasta
>
> **Roasted chicken** – pair with roasted potatoes, carrots, and beets with rosemary and sea salt
>
> **Mahi-mahi** – serve grilled, paired with mango-coconut chutney and stirfried veggies
>
> You can find the recipes for all these pairings in the resources section on our website.

vegetable intake was pretty low. I fell far short of the five-servings-a-day recommendation every single day.

But during those weeks, the box of produce became the starting point for my meals. Instead of asking what I could have with my Hamburger Helper (often nothing), I asked myself what would go well with beets, carrots, potatoes, tomatoes, and spinach.

A trip past the butcher counter to mix and match protein with my produce inspired food pairings that have stayed with me to this day – pork chops, spinach salad, and summer squash; beef stew with carrots and potatoes; collard greens, tomato salad, and fresh sausage, to name just a few.

Even after these weeks of new culinary adventures, I would often start my shopping trips in the produce section, buying what looked fresh and pairing great produce with my favorite sources of protein.

To this day, I tend to start my meal planning with one fresh ingredient and see where it takes me. It rarely leads me astray, and always ends with a day filled with more fresh food and fewer processed foods than the old Roland ever ate.

You don't have to be forced by circumstances (faced with a box of produce that will rot if not eaten) to build your own meals based on the freshest ingredients, but if you think it will help, order yourself a CSA basket and give it a try!

Your tasks for this chapter:

1. Spend this week exploring the wide variety of fresh vegetables that are available to you. Go for seasonal produce at your farmer's market or supermarket. Pick a favorite vegetable or two, and then pick a good protein source to go with it. There's no right or wrong, and you can refer to our food pairings above for ideas.

2. You can dive in headfirst by signing up for a CSA basket. You could be introduced to fruits and vegetables that you've never heard of, much less tasted. A weekly basket is a reminder that seasons and produce dictate what happens in the kitchen; it is pure wisdom from our ancestors turned inspiration for some of the most renowned chefs in the world.

3. Say no to packages for one week. Instead of processed or prepared foods from cans, packets, mixes, bottles, bags, jars, and boxes, start with fresh, raw ingredients from the produce section of your market or from your CSA basket. Prepare them

with love, spice them with passion, and enjoy wonderful meals inspired by the natural, fresh, and delicious food itself.

Where to next?

1. Eat Your Water (p.60)
2. Odds and Ends and the Anti-Cancer Soup (p.117)

19

Raw, Cooked, Juiced

by Galina

Oh, just eat your veggies!

We know we're supposed to eat plenty of fruits and vegetables, but we don't always think about why. Until we know that, it's hard to take. Why should you eat enough fruits and vegetables? Health is a complex topic, and providing the optimal environment for health is not easy. Some factors, like pollution, stress, having to work under artificial light, may not be controllable or modifiable. But food is a bit different, as you get to choose and influence what you eat.

Several studies show that increasing daily fruit and vegetable consumption to 600 grams (or a pound and a half) a day could "reduce the total worldwide burden of disease by 1.8%, and reduce the burden of ischaemic heart disease and ischaemic stroke by 31% and 19% respectively. For stomach, oesophageal, lung and colorectal cancer, the potential reductions were 19%, 20%, 12% and 2%, respectively."

Multiple scientific studies are showing that rich and varied consumption of fruits and vegetables could create an environment where we can prevent a large percentage of cancer, asthma, cardio-vascular disease, diabetes, and stroke from happening. While reading papers for our book, we stumbled upon a study showing a 50% decreased risk of oral cancer if one consumed fruits and vegetables.

The mechanisms are not yet well understood, but so far it's thought that the presence of anti-oxidants and phytochemicals fight free radicals, also known as oxidative damage, or aging of tissues. The macula in your eye is a great example of that – a yellow pigment called lutein, an anti-oxidant found in spinach, leafy greens, and carrots, protects this area. When the store of anti-oxidants – your fruit and veggie bank account – starts to run low, the area cannot rebuild and degeneration and loss of vision occurs. This process happens in different ways all over the body and at every stage of regeneration – imagine what that means to a skin cell, a liver cell, a gut cell, a pancreas cell. In one study, just one serving per day of leafy green veggies decreased the incidence of type 2 diabetes by 14%.

In a recent study I found to be super exciting, researchers even found that small additions of leafy green vegetables could dramatically improve the quality of blood, making it more diluted and improving blood flow to all areas of the body, preventing unnecessary clotting and possibly reducing the risk of stroke and heart attack. Exciting news!

Great! I am going to juice every day!

Before you go and buy a $599 blender and an annual pass to your local juice bar, consider the many benefits to *eating* your veggies, whether whole, raw, or cooked, versus consuming them blended, juiced, or extruded into a pill. A whole vegetable or fruit comes with fiber, and that slows down digestion and helps with elimination. Also, the process of chewing itself allows some of the carbohydrate to be broken down by enzymes in your saliva. Chewing also triggers the rest of the digestive system to release the necessary "juices" for that specific food's digestion.

I am not advising against juice or smoothies, but encouraging you to see them as a part of your fruit and vegetable intake, not a way to "check off" the fresh produce box in your daily menu. Liquid veggies and fruit, and juice in particular, are just not the same as whole produce.

Your gut bacteria – those microscopic colonies of hard-working organisms that make vitamins, ward off pathogens, and keep your blood sugar, hormonal, nervous, and immune systems in check, also need plenty of veggies to thrive. The fibers in your veggies are what those little guys feed on. Smoothies still have fiber, but it gets strained out when making juice.

Chewing also helps keep your teeth and jaw healthy. The teeth are supported by bone that needs stimulation, just like the bones in your legs, ribs, and spine need walking to thrive. Chewing is particularly of importance to kids whose bone structure is still developing – hand that toddler a carrot stick, not carrot juice; it will do him good.

The biggest bang for your buck

In *Eating on the Wild Side* Jo Robinson shares the fruit and vegetable challenge of today: Most fruits and vegetables have been so heavily modified to last long on the shelf that the natural content of phyto-nutrients – those same chemicals that should keep our cholesterol in check, fight infection, and make our eyesight sharp – has dropped to almost nothing.

She talks about a study where men were fed an apple a day to keep the doctor away, in this case to lower their cholesterol, yet the apple chosen for the study was so low in beneficial phytonutrients and so high in sugar that the men's triglycerides actually went up.

Her revolutionary book is a great tool to help us choose those plant varieties, both wild and domesticated, that give us the most health benefits. By following her simple charts, we've learned to easily opti-mize our fruit and vegetable choices, opting for varieties that have been shown to carry the most phytonutrients and anti-oxidants. This is also great news for those of us who are trying to maximize nutrition. You can get a lot of positive effects from produce with a few smart choices.

Here are some of the surprising and easy-to-implement tips we've incorporated from Jo Robinson's research.

Lettuce – Choose red leaf lettuce over green. When shopping for lettuce, opt for the open-leaf varieties, versus the ones that curl in a head with some of the leaves hidden from view. The more bitter, the better, so add some arugula, mustard greens, or endives to your salad mix. When you bring the lettuce home, wash and tear it in pieces. Store in a plastic bag that you perforate with a needle in several places. In the next day the anti-oxidant content of the lettuce will have increased.

Onion and garlic – Jo advises choosing the hotter and more pungent varieties of onions. Green onions, also known as scallions, are the most power packed of the onion family. Shallots, which are mild and flavorful, have six times more beneficial nutrients than the typical onion. To optimize the most beneficial quality of garlic, its allicin content, she advises you chop, mince, or press it, and then let it sit for 10 minutes before you use it – the time after cutting allows the allicin to develop. Heat can destroy allicin, so for best results add it at the end of cooking.

Potatoes, carrots, and beets – Jo's advice here is simple. Go for the more colorful varieties, including purple, yellow, orange, and eat the skin of the organic varieties. To reap all the benefits of beets, Jo says to cook the greens like you would spinach. Cooking improves the bioavailability of nutrients in both carrots and beets, so consider that the next time your raw-juicing friend tells you that you're killing your food by cooking it.

Tomatoes – Smaller and darker tomatoes pack more nutrients and flavor, so the darker the better. Tomatoes are another veggie that becomes even better for you if you cook it, releasing the potent anti-oxidant lycopene.

Crucifers – From broccoli and cauliflower to the ubiquitous kale, crucifers reign supreme on the pages of Jo's book. Kale, she says, is one of the few cultivated veggies that can compare to wild varieties of leafy greens. An important thing we learned from her is that broccoli loses a lot of its benefits when stored for even a short time. It's best to buy fresh broccoli at a farmer's market and eat the same day or soon after. Short cooking times are best for these veggies, with steaming and sautéing preferred.

Apples – Go for color, eat the skin, and opt for organic. Apples are one of the most pesticide-treated crops out there!

Berries – Strawberries tend to increase their anti-oxidant value if you pick them or buy them fresh, and then store them on the counter for a couple of days. It's best to eat wild berries, so if you live where they are available, make a point to go out and gather – wild berries have much higher levels of micronutrients than their cultivated counterparts. Eat frozen berries, too, as freezing preserves the nutrients well. Smaller berries, such as blueberries and blackberries, spoil fast, so if you can't eat them right away freeze them or cook them. I was surprised to find out that cooking can even increase the antioxidant capacity.

We've been paying close attention to Jo Robinson's advice for the last couple of years and it has guided what we grow on the patio. We currently have several varieties of red lettuce, chives, garlic, black and cherry tomatoes, and kale in our aeroponic Tower Garden. We just planted several different varieties of cherry tomatoes and black tomatoes. Our crop isn't huge, but what we do grow has maximum nutrition!

A note on microgreens and sprouts

A delicious and easy way to add nutrient-dense veggies to your diet is to incorporate microgreens – the baby plants of leafy greens, crucifers, and herbs. The microgreens of kale, broccoli, arugula, radishes, and basil contain several times the amount of anti-oxidants and microelements the older plants do. It differs by plant, but there can be up to 40 times more in a baby plant compared to full grown.

> **LEAFY GREENS AND THYROID DISEASE**
>
> Leafy greens and crucifers can contain compounds called goitrogens, which can inhibit the uptake of iodine by the thyroid gland. People suffering from thyroid disease should consult a nutritionist to make sure that they know how much is safe to consume, as well as how to prepare them to minimize the goitrogens.

You can easily grow microgreens yourself or buy them at farmer's markets and stores. The tiny plants add a lovely flavor to salads, and a gourmet touch to sandwiches and soups. Even picky eaters can add microgreens to smoothies and salads and easily reap the benefits without feeling like they have to eat bowls of greens.

One step further down in the growing process is sprouts. Sprouts are the seeds of plants that have been soaked and germinated. Sprouting greatly increases the availability of anti-oxidants and enzymes of the seed, and also improves digestibility. Once the tiny sprout pokes its head out, they are ready to enjoy, seed, root, stem, and all. You can sprout most common seeds, grains, and legumes yourself, or find them in the produce section of the market.

Our favorite ways to add more vegetable goodness

Breakfast: We add veggies to egg scrambles and frittatas or make a vegetable and fruit smoothie to go with breakfast. A cup of berries as a side is a great way to start your day with something both sweet and flavorful.

Our top breakfast veggies and fruits: We like scallions, mushrooms, spinach, kale, celery, sundried tomatoes, slow-roasted tomatoes, and sweet potatoes; green apples, bananas, plantains, pineapple, berries, lemons, and oranges.

Snacks: Fresh cut-up veggies and fruits, as well as dried veggies and fruits, are amazing snacks. I really enjoy dried broccoli and kale, and if you have a dehydrator at home you can make any dried veggies for easy and portable snacks.

Our top snack veggies and fruits: We like carrot and celery sticks, cucumber, raw cauliflower, dried broccoli and kale chips; bananas, apples, pears, peaches, cherries, dark grapes.

Lunch and dinner: The simple rule we follow is to make a salad or side from at least two vegetables and have at least two cooked vegetables. This way between lunch and dinner we can get a rich variety. Cooking can be as simple as steaming or as complex and long as slow roasting.

Our top lunch and dinner veggies and fruits: Our favorites are radishes, beets, carrots, bell peppers, cucumbers, microgreens, sweet potatoes, asparagus, artichokes, cabbage, eggplant, seaweed, fermented vegetables like sauerkraut and kimchi, berries, papaya, pineapple, melon, frozen cherries.

Your tasks for this chapter:

1. We invite you to include as many varieties of fruits and vegetables as you can in your meals. You can start slowly by just finding opportunities for one veggie per meal or one fruit per snack, until you become comfortable with the idea.

2. Try a recipe this week that *only* contains veggies and fruit. Ratatouille is labor intensive, yet rich and flavorful. Roasted mixed veggies are easy and accessible in every season.

3. Optional: Grab a copy of Jo Robinson's book at the library for a rich reference on the amazing benefits of selecting and properly preparing veggies and fruits.

Where to next?

1. Take the Eating-In Challenge (p.66)
2. Finding Your Fitness Path (p.186)

Just Look, You Don't Have to Touch

by Galina

20

Paying attention to your pee and poo can show you the path to optimal health

Not unlike a snowflake, each bowel movement has a uniqueness that should be regarded with wondrous appreciation. Too often dismissed as useless and malodorous waste, poo has struggled since the dawn of time to receive the respect it deserves.

— Josh Richman and Anish Sheth, *What's Your Poo Telling You*

There is nothing that reminds you that you are in a foreign land like the first encounter with a local restroom. And it's not just the bizarre water taps and the different ways you pull paper towels out of the dispenser. It's deeper.

On my first arrival to America, I was quite bewildered by the local toilet bowl. I thought there was something broken, since it was half full of water. I braved it anyway, and I ended up fine, my terror of toilet water splatter aside. A couple of years later I discovered that culture shock worked both ways.

Upon arrival to Eastern Europe, many of my American friends would rush out of the bathroom asking why the toilet had no water in it, and what the heck was the story with the "poop podium"? Some of the older style toilet bowls used to have a design that allowed bowel movements to hit a firm and shiny porcelain plateau, so you could view the miraculous works of your digestive system. Fantastic for hospitals, if the doctor wanted to run some diagnostics, yet quite possibly the last thing my Western friends wanted to see.

Why would anyone want to see their poop, they would ask? A paragraph into this chapter, you may be asking yourself the same thing. Why would you?

The digestive system, from mouth to anus, is 30 feet long. In the brilliant words of Mary Roach, author of *Gulp: Adventures on the Alimentary Canal*, "it is like the Amtrak line from Seattle to Los Angeles: transit time is about thirty hours, and the scenery on the last leg is pretty monotonous."

This unseen, dark, and enclosed world is the cradle of our health. It hosts the ingestion and assimilation of food, the creation of useful vitamins and fats, the killing off of harmful pathogens, the fragile balancing of our immune system, the production of hormones and neurotransmitters, as well as a large portion of our nervous system structures. Known as the "second brain" or the "enteric nervous system" the GI tract is home to 100 million neurons, more than the number in your spinal cord.

Health is not a static state. If anything it is a dynamic optimal scenario for the function of all systems and organs, the stage upon which life happens. But that dynamic scenario also has parameters that make it more or less optimal, each day. You may wake up with a headache one day, feel some stiffness in your ankle another. We have a baseline idea for the "feel good" states of most systems. When it comes to digestion, your poo and pee can tell you a ton about the state of the 30 feet of digestive tract, whose inner workings are hidden from the outside world. You can't sense the assimilation of nutrients, or the production of biotin, or serotonin, yet you can see in plain sight if you have a soft stool or if your pee looks foamy and cloudy. If you never look down there, how will you know what your baseline of "feel good" digestion is?

I asked my lovely friend, digestive and reproductive health specialist Barbara Loomis, to shine some light on digestion, and give us much needed advice that will help us understand, accept, and care for our digestion better.

Digestion is something hard to talk about. It seems difficult in our Western culture to discuss the "down there" subjects. Yet, this is what you do for work every single day!

As a manual therapist who works with the belly I'm super comfortable *and* fascinated by the inner workings of the bowels. I remember being intrigued as a kid as I sat on the toilet listening with a stethoscope to my guts in action. It's amazing to listen to all the activity going on inside...or at least I think so. Most people, however, flush and forget about it. People feel vulnerable when it comes to their bellies and what's inside. I get it, we're taught to conceal, cover up, not talk about, or ignore our inner workings. My goal is not only to help improve reproductive and digestive health, but also to help people restore their connection to their bodies and listen to the physical messages. The body knows, we just have to listen.

What does healthy digestion look like?

Healthy digestion is when all organs are working as a team. We should feel good after eating, and be free from excessive gas and bloating. Our stools should be well formed but soft, free from blood and mucus. If these substances appear, there's a problem. Acid reflux is another warning sign that things are amiss. Contrary to popular belief, acid reflux is often a sign of too *little* stomach acid. Yet most people think it means too much acid. When gastric acid is low, food sits in the stomach longer than it should, ferments, and gasses off.

The gas-filled stomach swells and pushes on the cardiac sphincter, the valve between the stomach and esophagus. Over time, this can create inefficiency in the sphincter causing acid to splash into the esophagus, which results in burning pain.

> **BARBARA'S 5 RULES OF GOOD DIGESTION:**
> 1. Don't eat on the run.
> 2. Don't overeat.
> 3. Don't eat in front of the TV or talk politics while you eat.
> 4. Smell your food.
> 5. Connect with your food.

It's hard to tell if you digested well today – where do you start?

Look at your poo. It is a clue to how your digestive system is functioning. "Soft serve" poo may be a signal of lactose intolerance. If your stools are not formed well and exit the body in pieces, this could indicate a sign of a lack of fiber. Fiber acts like glue in the colon to hold the stool together. Greasy, gassy, and smelly stools may be a signal that the liver and gall bladder are not functioning properly. Ideally, your stool should be golden brown and well formed.

At least one complete bowel movement in the morning would be ideal. If you're not eliminating daily, broken-down hormones and toxins that are in the colon may permeate through the intestinal wall into the bloodstream.

Other signs that digestion is not optimal may be evident from skin breakouts, gas and bloating, thyroid problems, fatigue, or other signs of malnourishment.

How do different organs play together in digestion?

The Western mind likes to break things down into parts, but the reality is that no one part of digestion works in isolation. Digestion actually starts in the brain, before you even put food in your mouth. This phase of digestion is called the cephalic (brain) phase. This cephalic phase is triggered by the sight, smell, and memory of food. Consider this: If we mindlessly shove food in our mouths while doing other things, like watching TV, we don't give our bodies a chance to prepare for the incoming food. It's like having an uninvited guest pop in unannounced.

What about urine? What do we look at?

Ideally urine should appear clear and light yellow. If your urine is foamy, it could be a sign of excess protein. Urine that smells sweet can indicate a blood sugar imbalance.

If someone was having digestive complaints, noticing unusual poo and pee or gas and bloating, or general feelings of stagnation and feeling stuck, what kind of a specialist should they reach out to?

It depends on the severity and underlying cause of the symptoms. Lab tests may be required to rule out a serious condition. As far as manual therapy goes, I would seek out someone trained in Visceral Manipulation™, or Chi Nei Tsang (Chinese abdominal therapy). Chi Nei Tsang encompasses massage, breath work, and Chi Kung principles. Visceral Manipulation™, developed by osteopathic physician Jean-Pierre Barral, incorporates gentle techniques that improve internal organ function by optimizing the organs' natural movement.

Since diet is foundational for proper digestive function, it's also important that individuals work with practitioners who can offer assistance in this area. A functional nutritionist, naturopathic physician, or someone specializing in nutrition would be a good choice. Nutrition science has come a long way in the last few years, so seeing someone who is up to date in their education and treats the individual as the unique complex being they are is crucial.

Are there any postural changes we can make?

Sitting throughout the bulk of the day is tough on the digestive system. Excessive sitting is a major contributor to constipation. This is especially true for sitting with a posteriorly tilted (tipped back) pelvis. This position puts your body in the shape of a C and everything between the pelvis and ribcage gets displaced. Several of my clients who have made the shift to dynamic workstations (workstations that keep them moving in a variety of positions) have been able to resolve their constipation issues.

How you position yourself during elimination is also important. Using a squatting platform or raising your knees up by putting a stack of books or yoga blocks under your feet can help to position yourself into a modified squat. This position allows the puborectalis, the sling-like muscle that wraps around the rectum, to relax. In addition, when you lean forward, hinging from the hips, not by flexing the spine or at the waist, the top of your femurs will press against your abdomen giving a lift and slight compression to the colon, making bowel movements much easier.

What about holding? Many people are bathroom averse and wait to go to the bathroom.

When you habitually ignore the urge to go poo, your pelvic floor and anal sphincter may become dysfunctional, and your rectum may become unresponsive. The rectum contains stretch receptors that signal when it's time to find a bathroom. If you ignore the signal, water gets pulled out of the colon and the stool dries out, making it more difficult to expel. Do this repeatedly and you may even over-stretch the colon, affecting its tone and ability to function properly.

What causes the sensation of bloating and things not moving through? People complain of not being able to close their pants. Is it all nutrition or is it more about organ and skeletal alignment?

I would say both. The sensation of bloating is caused by internal pressure, typically from gas. Causes of bloating could range from gut dysbiosis, improper diet, food sensitivities, stress, an overburdened liver, sitting too often and for long periods, poor skeletal alignment, and eating too fast or too much. With chronic overeating and poor structural alignment, the stomach can, over time, lose its tone, and the lower part of the stomach can droop down into the pelvis. This condition is called ptosis of the stomach and can cause flatulence, reflux, headaches after a large meal, rib and vertebral pain, heaviness after meals, and belching.

Tight clothing is often overlooked as a contributing factor to slug-gish organs. You may be following the fashion trends, but tight clothing can inhibit blood and lymph flow and place inappro-priate loads on the internal organs. Any kind of shape-wear (like super-constrictive undergarments) – or even the act of sucking in your stomach for extended periods – changes the pressures within the belly and interferes with proper flow and digestion.

Below are some tools to help you observe your own pee and poo and to assist you in starting your own digestion detective career.

First is the famous Bristol Stool Chart. Developed in the late 1990s, it helps identify seven different types of bowel movements, to give a smooth start to your detective work.

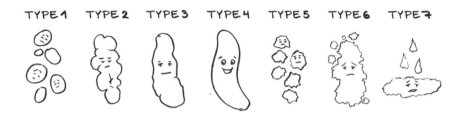

Type 1 – Separate hard lumps, difficult to pass, like rabbit poo. Those are typical in low-fiber diets, and also after treatments with medication that can cause a negative change in the natural gut flora.

Type 2 – Sausage shaped and lumpy. Shows constipation that has been going on for a while, and which can be potentially dangerous to the structure of the colon. Konstantin Monastyrsky warns that adding fiber will likely cause more issues to the person suffering from this type of jam.

Type 3 – Like a sausage with cracks in the surface. Slightly better than Type 2, but still showing signs of unhealthy poo, with lack of healthy flora and possibly a need to strain.

Type 4 – Like a sausage or snake, smooth and soft. This is your average healthy poo, with a circumference of 0.5 to 1 inch. It comes out easily and doesn't have a foul smell.

Type 5 – Soft blobs with clear-cut edges that pass easily. This may show a fast transit time.

Type 6 – Fluffy pieces with rugged edges and mushy stool. This type may show up after taking too many minerals, too much water, or indicate a hyperactive colon or bowel movements that are a result of stress.

Type 7 – Watery and no solid pieces. You have probably all seen diarrhea. And no, it's not normal.

What about pee?

Like Barbara said, above, healthy urine should appear clear and light yellow. Orange and amber urine typically indicate dehydration. Beets and certain medications can make your urine darker and unusual colors, but it can also indicate something more serious. If your urine smells sweet, is foamy or cloudy, or the color cannot be explained, see a doctor. It could be a sign of excess protein or sugar. You can check out a full-color urine chart on our website, at eatmovelive52.com.

How do you use all of this information? Well, how about you catalog it in your brain, under "down there" files? This way, once you have seen what "normal" is for you, it will be easy to spot an abrupt change.

Will you take the detective challenge? If you never look down there, how will you know what your baseline of "feel good" digestion is? If you never look, how will you ever know how you are doing?

Your tasks for this chapter:

1. Look down and see what your pee and poo look like. Take note of what is normal for you.

2. If you notice any signs of dehydration or food not fully digested, take simple steps, like drinking water and chewing your food thoroughly. If symptoms persist, see a doctor.

3. If you are struggling with digestive complaints and you feel like you have already done a lot with nutrition and stress management, but you are still constipated, have diarrhea, or irregular bowel movements, maybe it's time to research some therapists in your area. Those can be nutritionists or manual therapists who work with the digestive tract, like Barbara suggested above. We have links to websites that help you locate them in the resources at eatmovelive52.com

Where to next?

1. Eat Your Water (p.60)
2. What the Tooth? (p.325)

MOVEMENT AND EXERCISE

Walking Like Nature Intended   by Galina

21

In which you learn the elements of walking for health and longevity

I n our small community, you'll see many people out walking. One of the reasons is that the city planners built passages with carefully manicured landscaping between neighborhoods, wide and open sidewalks, and parks everywhere. This attracts a lot of active adults, who can be seen at sunrise and sunset, pumping away into the bright health horizon.

I teach walking classes weekly and one of our favorite places to go is a lake 1.1 miles around. This allows everyone to pace themselves, and choose if they want to walk a bit or a lot.

One of our exercises is observing everyone for what we call walking form. Watching someone's walking form is a very simple and easy way to get insight into the complex world of their gait mechanics. The body has 360 joints. With each step, each joint should experience movement – some of those movements are tiny and microscopic, but others, like the movements of your ankles, hips, and shoulders, are large and easy to spot.

When we look at walking form, we always want to watch for essential movements happening, the way they occur, and look for a way to encourage and find better movement from the inside out. This ensures that our body is functioning in a way that properly loads our systems – skeletal, muscular, cardiovascular, nervous, digestive.

Take something as simple as foot position. When you're out today, watch people walking and notice their feet.

Foot position determines how the ankle joint, knee, hip, sacroiliac

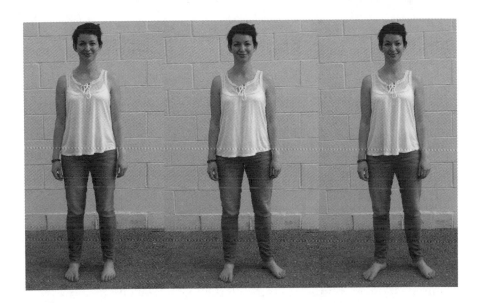

joint, spine, and shoulders will move during your gait cycle. Notice how people whose feet turn out lumber along versus gliding forward. Notice how someone whose ankles flex and move more is able to move forward through space in one beautiful motion, and someone whose ankles are tight is bouncing up and down and left and right.

Another component of walking form is arm swing – are the arms swinging front and back or left to right? In our computer-focused, chair-bound society, the shoulders often roll forward, and the tissues in the front of the chest tighten, drawing the arms forward and messing up our reflexes. It was once natural to swing the arms forward and back, but now, due to altered bone positions, many of us swing left to right.

Why is looking at walking form important? Well, most people walk for health, right? Most of my clients are walking for metabolic benefits – they hope to increase energy expenditure, burning more calories during the walk and after. If you have better walking form, you can actually better use the large muscles in your body and burn more calories. Walking is also a stress reliever, and the ability to walk smoothly and pain free is a great way to help stress melt away.

Another reason people walk is to keep the cardiovascular system functioning optimally – most people are well versed in walking to prevent high blood pressure and heart disease. That goal also requires that our body parts are moving in a way that helps return blood to the heart with every step. An efficient and natural gait translates to better blood flow throughout the body.

A third reason is maintaining bone mass – there are many studies showing the bone-building effects of walking. But to maximize these effects you need to be walking well. Optimally, your body should be aligned – from bottom to top – so that each tiny vibration from every little step sends a signal from your feet all the way up to your head, and to all the bones, muscles, and tissues in between. These little signals are what trigger bone strength and growth.

I mentioned stress earlier, and for good reason. Going for a regular stroll might help keep depression at bay. In a very cool study, only 10 days of walking was shown to improve the mood of people who had been depressed for an average of 6 months. There is no medication that promises these kinds of results!

Recently, Stanford University came out with a research report that examined walking and demonstrated its positive effects on creativity, associative memory, and ability to generate novel ideas. Score again, and the effects of creativity lasted even after the walk had been completed!

So here you are on your bone-building, blood pressure–lowering, calorie-incinerating, depression-busting, creativity-generating walk. What can you do now to ensure you are walking with good form? Glad you asked!

Walking should be a natural activity, but as you know from previous chapters, our civilized world has done a number on our "natural" functions. You can be a better walker – making sure your cardiovascular system is optimally aligned for the task, bones are supporting you in the right places, and you are using the big muscle groups to their maximum potential – with just a few simple alignment rules. You will see with practice that "backing your hips up" and allowing your pelvis to stack on top of your legs will let you use your glutes, hamstrings, and back muscles more, and better, than before!

It starts with the pelvis

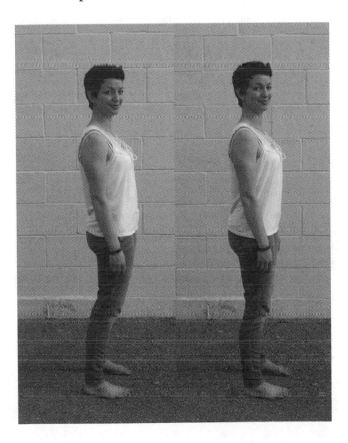

The first part of your body you want to adjust is your pelvis. Make sure that your pubic bone is not in front of the body. When your pelvis is "tucked" that leads to changes in the position of the femur bones and then your whole lower leg ends up pointed out, too, and then you are walking like a duck.

Bring the pelvis back behind you, with the tailbone free from the confinement of the meaty glutes, so that the pelvis stacks right on top of femur bones. Then when you walk, they can be free to move back and forth – into extension and flexion, on their natural trajectory.

Then move on to the feet

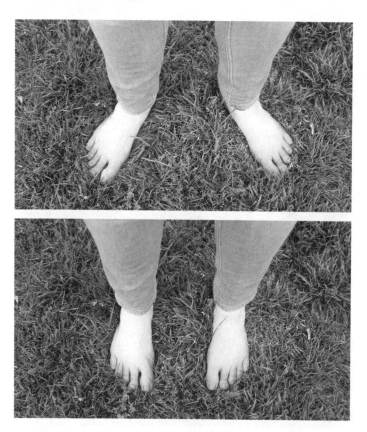

EAT WELL, MOVE WELL, LIVE WELL

To the best of your ability, point your feet straight. If you tend to be a very narrow walker, space your feet slightly apart, so that your feet are directly under your hip joints. As you walk, do your best to point your feet straight. Do not attempt to do that before you have untucked your pelvis. If you still find it challenging to walk with feet straight, take slightly smaller strides and give yourself time with our foot mobilizing exercises.

Align the ribcage

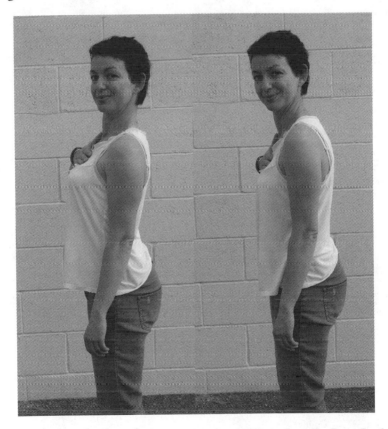

Maybe you tend to slouch when you walk, or maybe you look like you are in the military – chest high and proud! If you place a hand on your sternum, it should be closer to vertical. The ribcage itself should sit directly over the pelvis. As you walk, this will allow the muscles of your torso to participate fully, and will ensure ample space for breathing.

Let the arms swing

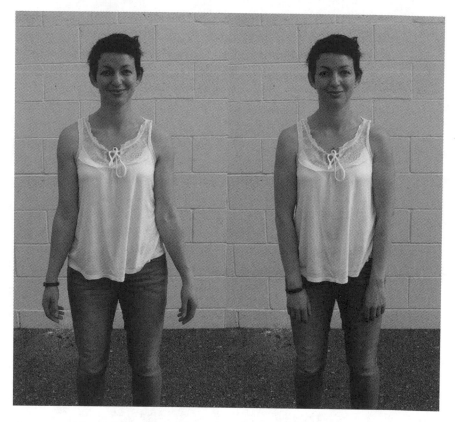

As you walk and one leg is swung in front of you, the same side arm swings backward. That reflex-driven motion is an important part of stabilizing the spine while not allowing excessive twisting and bending. In order for your arms to swing well, the upper arm bone – your humerus – needs to be facing straight. To make sure that it is, allow the elbow pit to face forward and your arms to swing freely at your sides.

Head over shoulders

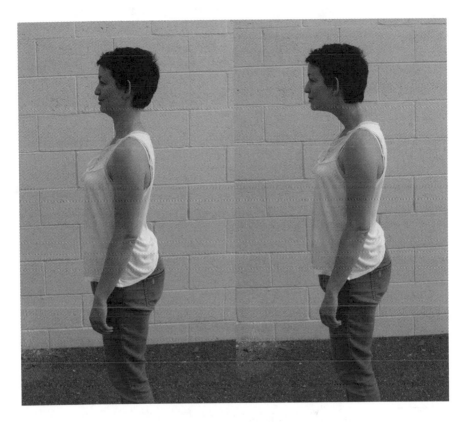

If you watch people walking, you will see that the majority have their heads jutted way out in front of them. In proper walking alignment the ears should be directly over the shoulders, allowing for an effortless balance of the head and optimal positioning of your airway, esophagus, and the major blood vessels passing through the neck.

Now let's put it all together – pelvis back, feet straight, ribcage over pelvis, arms swinging, and head over the shoulders.

These elements take a while to master – in fact even my most advanced students only work on one or two of them as they walk. The great news is that even working on one of them can greatly influence the alignment of the rest of the body and help you get stronger bones, healthier blood vessels, leaner muscles, and improved mood. And while you are out for your walk, you may get a new creative idea! Head over to our website to share it with us!

Your tasks for this chapter:

1. This week and month, take short walks focusing on one of the elements above – working on walking form one element at a time. Start with the feet and pelvis, add the ribcage, head position, and arm swing. Each of those can be worked on separately or you can mix and match. Maybe for the first few minutes of your walk you work on your feet and then switch to other elements.

2. As you progress in later weeks, adding the rest of the elements, try to envision your body as being lighter and hanging up from the sky – the skeleton gracefully moving forward and gliding through each heel strike. Notice the slight spiral movements of the spine, the powerful push off the back of the body, the arms swinging opposite to the legs.

3. Once you have mastered the elements, find even more ease in your walk. Could you land slightly softer on your heel, could you hold less tension in the knee as the straight leg in front contacts the ground?

If you become truly interested in walking form, there are many schools to help you continue your education. You can head over to NutritiousMovement.com to find a teacher in your area, or look up Feldenkrais Method and Alexander technique practitioners. As always, take your time, be gentle with yourself, and let your body adapt to the changes one step at a time.

For a full list of resources for this chapter, head over to eatmovelive52.com

Where to next?

1. Meet Your Feet (p.164)
2. Drink Coffee. Not Too Much. Mostly Black. (p.95)

Meet Your Feet

by Galina

22

Fix your feet from the ankles down

L ike any machine meant to transport us over the Earth, the human body has a point of contact with the ground. You're probably familiar with the way your car works – tires contact the ground, translating the force up through the mechanism of the wheels and transmission to propel the whole body of the car forward and take you on a romantic road trip or on a late-night run for ice cream.

Human feet are our own tires – that point of contact with the surface, which propels us forward, up, sideways, or backward. The condition of your tires determines how your car feels on a bumpy or icy road, and the same with your feet – the condition of your feet and their mobility determines how well they serve the whole machine.

Foot pain and conditions like plantar fasciitis are obvious signs of a problem, but not every sign is so obvious. Some other indicators that your feet may be starting to fail you are loss of balance, tripping easily or often, losing your ground when you are in a hurry, or rolling and spraining your ankles.

Outward symptoms may vary from swelling to bunions to hammertoes, calluses, and corns. Pain in your knees, ankles, hips, and low back may also originate way down in the foot. Maybe you are comfortable in heels, but going barefoot is killing you? Do you often get cold feet? Did your doctor diagnose plantar fasciitis or neuroma? Does running practically destroy your shins?

I'm only asking because a lot of these conditions and symptoms

EAT WELL, MOVE WELL, LIVE WELL

are considered "normal." As normal, they can be discounted, overlooked, and simply put up with, often needlessly.

While they may be normal to you, as in your-grandma-had-them normal, they do not *normally* occur if you have good foot mobility and health, just like heart disease doesn't normally occur in a healthy cardiovascular system.

What causes our feet to lose their nature-given ninja status? For one, our shoes. There is also our overall lack of movement, plus a lack of interesting, varied, untamed-by-man walking surfaces. Go out in nature, walk on different paths, climb up trees, and your feet and toes will get way more exercise than what they do on a stroll in the nearby mall or on a concrete sidewalk. Our feet are amazing, but like any amazing machine, they won't do much if the environment does not require it or allow it.

It's safe to say that most of us can benefit from perfecting the mobility, foot posture (yes, your foot has a posture), and performance of our feet, because there is huge room for improvement there. However, it's not as simple as taking off your shoes and throwing them away! Just like removing the cast from a broken and healed limb, removing the shoe from a foot that has been bound in it since the age of one or two will require that you take things slowly. You will need to see what your foot is capable of today, and then retrain it to do what it has lost the ability to do.

Let's inspect your feet.

What did you find on the little treasure hunt south of your ankles?

A bunion – Also known as hallux valgus. This deformity appears as we lose the strength in our foot and the whole limb collapses onto the inside of the ball of the foot with every step you take. Think of

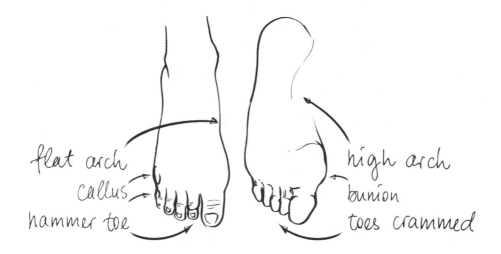

flat arch
callus
hammer toe

high arch
bunion
toes crammed

it this way: instead of moving back behind you in one straight, clean line, the leg rolls in and the mechanical forces of gait slam that poor bone into the ground. The body eventually ends up building extra tissue to protect the foot and the abnormal joint. That tissue is the bunion. Often, a bunion begins with shoes that sport a toe box that's too tight, a front that is lifted too high or a positive heel, then later continues to be formed and deformed by the forces of gait.

Hammer toes – The four smaller toes of the foot sometimes get stuck in extension – where one joint is pulled up by tension in the lower leg. That often starts as the toes are being crammed into too small or narrow a shoe or sock, or by the muscular action of grabbing on to a flip-flop. Whatever the source of your hammer toes, you need a movement program to address them. Oh yes, and throw out your flip-flops too! At the very least, save them for the gym shower and short trips like taking out the garbage.

Calluses and corns – Those guys show up when your shoes rub against your skin, creating pressure and friction. The body responds by laying down extra skin, but then the raised surface itself becomes another place to press and rub against. If you have these, know that they will not go away and stay away until you remove the shoe that is constricting them. There's a list of great minimal shoes in the resources section for this chapter at eatmovelive52.com.

Toes too cramped together – Remember how spread out the Flintstones' feet were? Your toesies are naturally supposed to have some space between them. That allows the metatarsals to meet the phalanges in good alignment, ensuring pain-free and smooth transition over all 33 joints of the foot. Narrow shoes change that arrangement. The forefoot becomes almost unusable (and unused), and cramped toes with tons of pressure placed upon them are an injury waiting to happen. This may manifest as hammertoes, bunions, neuromas, or, later on, as low back pain, possibly even contributing to a hip fracture.

Flat feet or pancake feet – You don't need to have Arc de Triomphe (do you like my French?) arches to function well. However, if your whole foot contacts the floor and you see that the medial malleolus (those are the round boney knobs on your inner ankle) are taking a steady dive inward and toward the floor, then some foot strengthening is in order. Those feet may also look loose and sloppy, and roll in when walking.

Arch too high and rigid – Now if you *do* have Arc de Triomphe arches, that may mean that your foot is too rigid and stiff to function well. People with rigid and high arches usually tend to hang out on the outside of the foot and have a hard time creating stability through the front of the foot. Less of the sole of the foot reaches the ground, so there is less surface area available to stabilize yourself and push yourself off the ground when you walk.

Now test the mobility and strength of your toes. You should be able to move each toe at will. Can you lift your big toe without lifting the other four, or excessively forcing them into the ground? Can you lift the small four toes without lifting the big toe? Can you spread your toes out and away from each other? Can you squeeze them together?

There are numerous small yet indispensably important muscles in your feet that all need stimulation. Tiny muscles in your feet called interossei and lumbricals work hard to move the joints in your feet whenever you're upright. We expect them to support and control our full bodyweight like a monster truck's tires do, even as we expect them to give us the agility of a sports car. It's the ability of your toes to move well that keeps them and your feet healthy, strong, and agile, so the next time you trip playing Frisbee you won't end up in an ankle brace. The more mobile the joints in your feet are, the more information the foot can relay up to the brain, giving the rest of your muscles the ability to react appropriately to the challenges!

If you are having a hard time moving your toes like in the exercises above, then you are also deprived of the full capability to relay important information from the ground up to your brain, and unfortunate compensations up the chain can occur. When your hip lifts on one side every time you walk, it could be because your big toe didn't bend to allow forward movement, for instance.

So where do you start when it comes to recovering your foot shape and strength? There are many simple exercises you can do anytime throughout your day to improve your feet, so let's get started!

Your tasks for this chapter:

1. Stretch your calves in the morning.

Grab a towel and roll it up to the thickness of a wine bottle and put it in front of you. Space your feet hip-width apart. Step forward and place one foot at the edge of the towel, keeping the foot straight. Walk forward with the other foot until you feel a stretch in the calf of the front foot. Keep the pelvis from rotating and do not bend at the waist! Keep weight in the heel of the stretching leg and both legs straight. You can step forward or back to adjust the amount of stretch. Hold for a minute on each side and repeat several times.

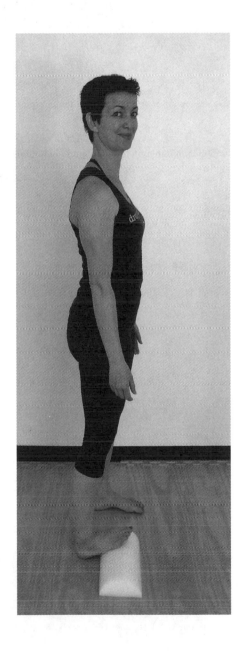

2. Stretch your toes

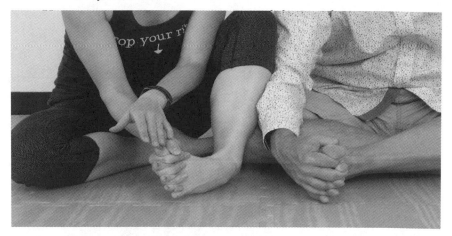

You can also passively stretch your toes while resting or sleeping – with a pair of toe separators, such as Correct Toes, or toe stretch socks, such as Happy Feet socks. Wear them for a few minutes at first to all through the night as you progress. Correct Toes can even be worn while walking in minimal shoes – score!

3. Massage your feet

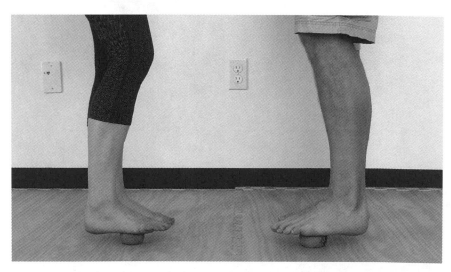

Use a tennis ball to massage your feet daily. Place it directly under your foot and roll back and forth, focusing on releasing tighter, stickier spots. Don't use too much weight. It should feel good.

It takes time to recover your foot health after years of covering them in shoes and walking on manufactured and manicured ground. Ultimately, your shoes need to change as much as your feet, but giving your feet some tender loving care is a great start.

Restoring your foot health may take longer for some of you, especially if your foot treasure hunt revealed more than you bargained for. Start small. Every day this week, do one of the drills above – from massage to stretching to spreading the toes or even using toe separators. Rediscover your connection to your feet and let us know how you're doing!

Where to next?

1. Level Up Your Vacation (p.284)
2. Something Fishy This Way Comes (p.102)

23

Take off Your Shoes

A Borneo story

I've always had super wide feet, and as a pre-internet kid it made shoes that fit really hard to find. When I was a little boy, my father worked on a long-term project overseas, so my family and I got to go and live on the tropical island of Borneo. Somehow, on one of the many layovers en route to the island, I lost my one pair of shoes! It was impossible to find shoes in Borneo that fit me, and as I wouldn't wear flip-flops, I took to going barefoot everywhere. At first it was a little tough, but after a few weeks I was running, jumping, and, in my mom's words, "walking over broken glass" in my bare feet.

Lucky me!

My feet got to spend a year away from the sensory deprivation chambers that we call shoes. My feet got to grow as nature intended, and grow they did; bigger, stronger, and more nimble. After my barefoot year, my feet were tough and strong, and I was faster than the neighborhood kids were in their sneakers.

But, when I got back to America, I got new shoes. They hurt. The only EEE shoes available were hard, stiff, expensive, ugly, and often orthopedic. So I chose to squeeze my quickly growing triangles into more "normal" shoes – I had to buy shoes two sizes larger just to get into them, and forgot about any extra space beyond my toes.

Within a year, my feet started to take on the shape of my narrow shoes. My toes were now angled in, coming to more of a point, my pinkie toe got pushed under the next little piggy, and I grew a pointed, painful callus that constantly caused me issues. The elevated heels of my cross-trainers and running shoes, recommended by my doctor for my "short calves," over time made my calves even shorter.

Soon, I'd lost many of the benefits of having lived a year shoeless; my feet were once again sensitive when I was barefoot, which wasn't very often anymore. My calves were tighter and shorter, my arches dropped, and my feet got tired and sore when I went barefoot for more than a few minutes at a time. It was a vicious circle: the more I wore shoes, the more I had to wear shoes. The same thing has probably happened to you.

Are you ready to learn something new?

Sit down and take one shoe off, but only one.

That's right, take it off! How does that feel? If you're anything like me, what you feel is ahhhh, relief! But if you pay close enough attention, you might also notice that your foot *hurts*. Normally at this time you'd kick the other shoe off, put up your feet, or walk around the house a bit, distracting yourself as the pain slowly fades away. But don't!

Ready for the second shoe?

Take it slow.

Most shoes are pretty snug, and buckled or laced tightly onto your feet. Without actually taking your second shoe off, unfasten or untie it. Use your fingers to loosen the laces and spread the upper a bit. Notice how your foot feels right now. I doubt you can actually feel the blood supply returning to your foot, but that's what's happening right now. No, the blood wasn't totally stopped, but it was restricted, and along with it, the flow of oxygen and nutrients to the feet was restricted, as was the flushing of toxins and waste products from the area.

Now take the shoe off and toss it aside

Resist any urge to rub your foot. Instead spread your toes, wiggle them, curl them, and extend them. Most people will notice that their toes all move as one; all five toes clench or spread together. At this point, you'll probably feel a rush of warmth to the feet. There's that blood supply returning to the toes! Good. If you have socks on, now is the time to take them off, too.

Look at your feet

How do they look? Are they a traditional foot shape like you'd see in a comic or cartoon?

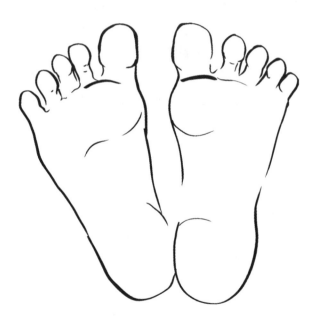

Or are they more shoe shaped?

How are your toes? Take your big toe, for instance. It should be pointing straight ahead, and in line with the inside edge of your foot. Is it? Or is it angling in toward your other toes?

Is your big toe pressed into your other toes, and pointing inward,

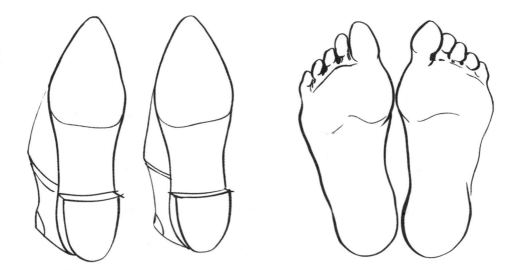

forming more of a shoe shape than a foot shape?

Do you have calluses where your shoe presses against your toes?

Is your little toe pushed underneath its neighbor?

Do you have bunions?

Ingrown toenails?

All of these little niggling things that cause pain in our feet are related to our shoes.

Time to stand up

But don't just stand up like you do every day. Pay close attention to the feeling in your feet as you stand up and put that first weight on your unbound feet. For me, it's a combination of pain and pleasure; like a back massage that hits just the right spot, only sometimes that right spot is a knot of painful, bound-up muscle!

After this feeling has fully sunk in, take a few small steps, and enjoy the sensation of carpet, wood, or tile that you might never have noticed because of the previously lingering pain. Feel free to sigh if you want to.

ARE BUNIONS GENETIC?

by Galina

Women often come to me complaining of bunions. When I ask them about their shoes, they tell me it's not their shoes, but genetic. "My mom and grandma had bunions, too."

One lady went so far as to tell me she is from Croatia and that all Croatians have bunions.

Sure, you might have a genetic predisposition to bunions, but it's not like going bald, or gray, or having blue eyes. You have a bunion because your shoes are forcing your feet into a position that creates a bunion, making you walk in a way that creates a bunion, and exercise in a way that creates a bunion. If you had the chance to move without the restriction of shoes, experience nature and an appropriate amount of movement, you'd probably never have a bunion. Perhaps your choice of shoes is genetic, too?

I'm the lucky one?

I think that my year of living shoeless helped in ways that I'm still benefiting from today. First, I remember how great my feet felt during that year of no shoes. Actually, I only remember because of the pain I started to feel when I was "lucky" to get shoes again.

Second, my feet had a whole year to develop during their critical growing period. Feet, like the roots of a plant, grow to fill the container in which they live.

As an adult, I've started to go barefoot as often as possible. Sure, my feet aren't growing anymore, but that doesn't mean I should keep them in a container. There are 19 muscles, 26 bones, 33 joints, and over 100 ligaments in the tiny space of your foot. All of those things are meant to be flexing and moving freely whenever you walk or run; not compressed and restricted by a shoe.

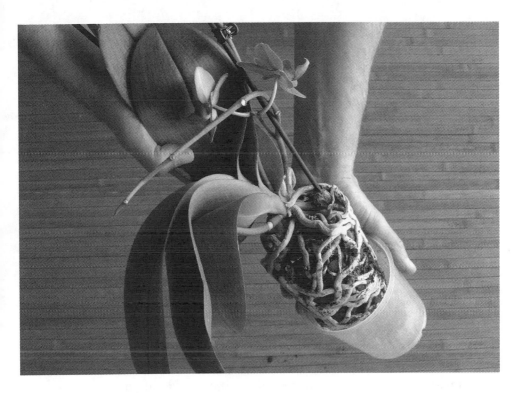

Feet contain over 200,000 nerve endings, and are an important part of the complex network of information-gathering, telling you where and how to move. You might have heard the term "proprioception" before? It refers to the awareness and perception of one's position in relation to the things around us. A shoe restricts that by forming a barrier between our foot and the rest of the world.

When you take off your shoes you get both short- and long-term benefits. In the long run, better proprioception leads to better movement, and better movement leads to *more* movement.

Movement done better

More movement, with better movement quality, leads to many long-term benefits, including better balance and increased confidence in one's own ability to move, which in turn leads to a decreased risk of falling, a lower chance of fractures, and a more independent life in later years.

By taking off your shoes, you allow your feet to move like nature intended, and take a load off your ankles, knees, back, and neck. Some conditions that seem far from foot health, like pelvic floor disorders and migraines, may well be rooted in your shoe choice.

If you are an athlete, you may greatly benefit from improving your foot mobility, which will help you ground and explode better for squats, lunges, jumps, and sprints.

Set your feet free

Take off your shoes when you get home!

Yes, it seems obvious, but you'd be surprised how many people leave their shoes on from morning until night, only taking them off when they get ready for bed. To remind yourself to take them off, set up an area at the front door where you can take off your shoes as soon as you get home.

Stop wearing slippers in the house

Although slippers are rarely as constricting as shoes, they still provide too great a barrier between your feet and the floor. If your feet are cold, wear socks, even if you need socks with grippy dots on the bottom. Yes, they do have them for adults (check eatmovelive52.com).

Errand shoes

If you need to go in and out of the house after you get home, a pair of slip-on loafers is handy to have around. Just don't get into the habit of leaving your shoes on all the time.

Hard floors?

If you have a kitchen with hard floors, like wood or tile, then standing to cook and clean can be fatiguing. A slip-resistant mat or rug can help during your transition from fully shod to shoeless.

Take it slow

You don't have to transition to living shoeless overnight.

If you are always in shoes, try to go barefoot or in socks for a few hours a day at first, then slowly transition to longer periods, until you can do it all the time.

You can do some of this in the house, but also outside in your yard, at the beach, at the park.

Discomfort means you are going too fast and you need to take a few steps back. Listen to your body and pay attention to the signals.

A foot exercise to rock your world

We teach our clients that stretching the calves is like brushing your teeth and flossing. It's so powerful that you'll find it in several chapters of this book, and it's described fully in our Meet Your Feet chapter.

Katy Bowman, author of *Simple Steps to Foot Pain Relief*, says that the calf stretch is the biggest bang for your buck exercise you will ever do as part of a daily routine.

Stretching your calves daily will help ease you into a life where your feet once again love their barefoot time!

> **LET YOUR KIDS GO BAREFOOT**
>
> Yes, one day they'll have to wear shoes, but until that day, let their feet grow naturally, get strong, and keep the mobility and dexterity that they were born with and meant to have.

Your tasks for this chapter:

1. Take off your shoes and get familiar with the structure of your feet. Commit to spending some time barefoot every day.

2. Notice how different surfaces feel on your feet over time – walk on carpet, sand, tile, grass. It can take a while for your feet to get used to pebbles and rocks, but it will come!

3. Stretch your calves. Remember the calf stretch from Meet Your Feet? Be sure to incorporate the calf stretch into your daily routine. In the morning, for sure, but for best results, stretch your calves several times per day.

Where to next?

1. I Have Needs (p.390)
2. Squat Your Way to Health (p.239)

Goodbye, Turkey Head

by Galina

24

A story of headaches and heartaches

The next time you go to a coffee shop, look around and check out people's postures.

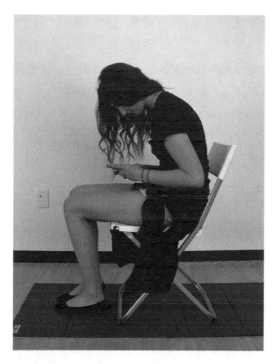

It's common to see a head that is jutted way forward, very much like an angry turkey. No big deal, you may say, since our body is so well adapted to various degrees of movement and ranges of motion – you can look up at the stars, down at your feet at the beach, behind you in the car. But when you habitually spend hours and hours with your head jutted in front of you, sooner or later, that catches up with you.

My studio is in a cervical care clinic, so I see many people with neck pain, migraines, jaw pain, and the associated syndromes. In scientific studies, neurovascular and musculoskeletal dysfunction (in plain English, nerve, vessel, muscle, and skeletal issues) are often correlated with the way we choose to hold our head relative to our shoulders.

The head and neck area are home to a number of vital systems. Your orientation system – balancing, hearing, and vision – depend on the optimal positioning of your eyes and ears, relative to your body and also relative to the ground. Large arteries pass through the neck. Cranial nerves exit the head and reach for the rest of the body. Your sense of smell, the function of your glands, your ability to produce speech, balance when walking, even feeling the touch of a loved one – depend on those nerves.

How you hold yourself affects your musculoskeletal system as well. Once your head starts to travel forward, the weight of it starts to pull your body forward. The muscles in the back of the neck and spine are soon working overtime and extra hard to keep the delicate functions within your neck and head from being interrupted. Over time, these compensatory movements create their own host of problems – artery hardening, migraines, snoring, and syndromes of the jaw. Our bodies function best in the positions they were meant to be in – just like the plumbing in your home – that is, straight and unkinked.

Postural neck pain is very common, and highly studied. One such study, looking at the relationship between posture and pain, found that subjects with more severe postural abnormalities experienced more frequent pain and discomfort. Another study looked specifically at standing. The more forward head posture young subjects had in standing, the more neck pain they experienced. Even wearing glasses, wearing them incorrectly, or choosing not to wear them when necessary can contribute to neck and upper back pain, as people often try to get closer to what they are looking at to see it more clearly. This tends to draw the head forward, down, or both.

In short, "backing your head up" can save you a lot of headaches, pun intended.

How do you know if you need to back your head up?

- You often find yourself jutting your head forward to read a book, listen to a friend talk, or read your computer monitor.
- You have asked someone to take a side shot of you and you see that your ear is not over your shoulder.
- You have tender spots, tightness, trigger points, in your upper back and shoulders.
- You have frequent headaches, snoring, TMJ syndrome, shortness of breath, sinus infections, thyroid disease, high blood pressure, hearing or vision loss.
- ...Or, you feel like an angry turkey.

No, seriously, if you are not sure of your head position the best way is to have a friend of family member take a picture of you while you are deep into a project – in front of a computer is a great chance, but books, TV, eating dinner will also do.

Now for the easy part. Take a seat with your spine tall. Tuck your chin back so that your ear is straight over your shoulder. Take a deep breath in through your nose. Now out.

While you try to get the hang of this, treat your neck as if it were made of something precious, like crystal – bring your head back with the least amount of effort necessary, and never force it. This would be a great time for your friend to take another picture for comparison!

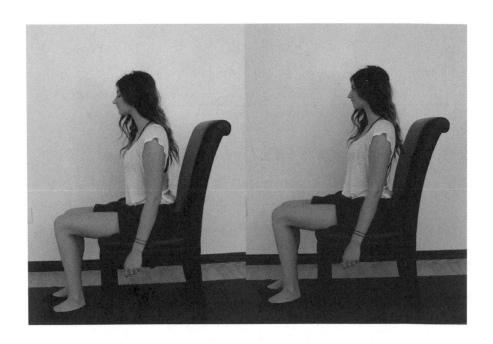

Your tasks for this chapter:

1. Have a friend or family member snap a photo of you when you're not looking. Preferably at work or when you are in your most focused posture. Notice if your head is forward.

2. Start to correct your head posture. Set a reminder on your phone or computer calendar to check your neck every couple of hours. Remember, it's just for a week. If you find that habit works for you, keep it.

3. After at least a week, and for as long as you feel like you need to work on this, have your friend take pictures of you working.

Enjoy your progress, and the lack of pain from your long gone turkey neck!

Where to next?

1. Roll With It (p.230)
2. Detox Your Pantry (p.44)

25 Finding Your Fitness Path

by Roland

There's no perfect fitness plan, just the perfect plan for YOU

There is no perfect exercise plan. Ideally, you'd be moving all day, every day, in nature. We might be meant to move, to lift heavy things, to jump, to swim, and to run, but the reality is that we are supposed to do those things simply as part of life. Civilization has seen to it that we no longer *have* to do them, and to make up for it, we invented exercise to keep ourselves "fit." Exercise fads come and go, whether it's the muscular strongman's body (think Arnold Schwarzenegger), the lithe runner's body, or the bendy yogi's physique. Yet none of these "fit" bodies is actually required for good health.

So, what IS important for good health?

If you look at your physical health as a byproduct of the natural environment, one where you would have spent most of your time migrating, looking for food, preparing it, and protecting it from others, sharing social responsibilities such as taking care of kids and your living spaces, then your "shape" or "physical health" is the outcome of everything you do merely to live your life.

You live life and shape happens. Bones get strengthened through walking, muscles get loaded carrying food or babies, your head stays in alignment because you are using it to transport objects. (When's the last time you carried something on your head?)

Essentially, this is what we are trying to mimic through exercise – those same benefits we would have gotten through natural movement. What are they?

Bone density – Diet, sunlight, and vitamin D are all important here, but bone density also comes from resistance training and even merely walking with good form. Our bones build density in response to the little shocks encountered during daily exercise and movement, vibration, and the pull of gravity, which is why good alignment and posture play a role.

Lean body mass – Lean body mass is bone, muscle, and things like tendons and ligaments. Pretty much everything *but* body fat. A good amount of LBM is a sign of good health. You don't have to have huge muscles, but studies do show that those with more lean body mass can weather the storms of illness, especially as we age.

Strength – Having strength lets you move more easily, walk more readily, and fall more skillfully, and hopefully without breaking a limb. Of course, it also comes in handy around the house, whether it's bringing in the groceries or carrying your child up to bed. In emergencies, like having to carry an injured friend down from a hike, strength is literally a life-saving quality. Once, we all possessed enough strength to live life and endure its emergencies. Now, we ask for help at the grocery store, because sometimes even a watermelon is too much to carry.

Alignment – Think of your alignment like you'd think of a car's alignment. If everything is lined up properly, you are more fuel efficient, more powerful, and the tires last longer. If your tires and wheels aren't in alignment, it's hard to drive fast, smoothly, and safely, much less drive for a long time without replacing parts.

Tissue quality – Technically, our body is made up entirely of tissues, but when we talk tissue, we tend to mean the softer stuff:

muscles, tendons, ligaments, fascia, and even skin. Tissues get micro levels of damage on a daily basis, and when we rest they recover, maintaining their size, elasticity, and hydration, or get stronger. With healthy tissues, we can move with better quality, recover efficiently from moving or exercising, get stronger, and feel energized after physical effort. Having achy muscles and joints, or being prone to spraining ligaments and straining tendons, or being tired and swollen after physical activity are all signs that you need to look at the quality of your movement, alignment, nutrition, rest, and stress levels. Pushing through a marathon only to get knee surgery after is not a sign of health (sorry!).

> **LEAN BODIES NOT REQUIRED**
>
> Did you know that being super lean is not ideal from a health standpoint? …Even if abs do look pretty hot!
>
> Studies have shown that a little extra weight is actually better for longevity. There are many theories as to why, but one is that the extra mass can give you the ability to better fight off disease. Extra weight, whether it's muscle or fat, is extra energy stored in your body for when you might really need it.

Cardio – Cardiovascular health is often talked about as if it's the be-all and end-all of fitness, but as you can see here, there's more to it than that. Still, good cardiovascular health is important for long-term health and quality of life. Good cardio comes from time spent not just in that mythical fat-burning zone, but at every range, from at rest, to walking, running, and all the way up to where your heart is pounding from a sprint or vigorous weight lifting session. When it comes to cardio, more is not always better. Studies show that overachievers (too much) are as at risk for heart failure as sedentary people (too little). As it is with the three bears, the goal with cardio is to be just right.

The minimum effective dose (yes, less can be more)

Our friend Dr. Mike T. Nelson is a PhD in Exercise Physiology, an exercise researcher, and a coach to athletes and regular Joes alike. Mike's specialty is studying exercise limits and effects via Heart Rate Variability, or HRV. HRV is a fancy measurement of heart rate and its consistency, which is affected not only by fitness levels, but stress levels, as well. HRV tells us a lot about whether a trainee or client is doing the right amount of exercise for them, not enough, or too much.

Measuring HRV helps assess fatigue, reaction to different modes and durations of exercise, as well as how your life and exercise combine to create positive or negative responses in the nervous and cardiovascular systems.

While many people do need to do more, you might be surprised to learn that it doesn't take as much as you'd think to get the health benefits of exercise. Mike says that when it comes to the question of how much exercise is best, the answer for many of us is "a little more than what you're doing today."

SHOULD YOU MEASURE YOUR HEART RATE VARIABILITY?

Many people have high levels of stress at work and at home and look to their exercise as a way to blow off steam. This can actually be the opposite of what you need. Exercise, particularly higher intensity or long duration cardio, is just another type of stress to the body. Adding more can lead to more damage, not better health. If you're not ready to invest in an HRV system right now, you can monitor your resting heart rate over time, and if you notice it starts to go up, look for ways to decrease the stressors on your system. Which areas of your work and home life are piling up? Tackle those first, whether it's lack of sleep, long hours, late nights, poor nutrition, or family matters. Working out more to reduce stress is probably not the answer.

Most people don't have an exercise or movement habit today, and suggesting that they go from sedentary, or close to it, to exercising five or more hours per week is a plan destined to fail. A sedentary person needs to first get up and walk, then walk farther, then a little farther. After that, we can talk about building the perfect plan, but even then, habits take time to build. Take your time, and know that just by doing a little better, you're actually doing *much* better.

We asked Mike (or Dr. Nelson, if you prefer) where he starts clients off when it comes to a new program, and lucky for us, Mike, Galina, and I all pretty much agree on the hierarchy of exercise!

You gotta walk before you can run

Walking is both underrated and overrated, depending on who you're asking. Doctors tell people to get out and walk, as if weight is going to melt off. Meanwhile, many personal trainers tell us that walking is a waste of time from a calorie burn perspective. It also doesn't raise your heart rate much, which is what many in the fitness business think cardio is all about.

What if I told you that both are right and both are wrong, but that it doesn't even matter?

Walking is first about health, not the calorie burn. Walking can bring improvements in heart health, insulin sensitivity, blood sugar, and appetite control, all of which can lead to a longer life and to the weight loss you're after. In fact, when it comes to what we typically want from our cardio – heart health – walking can be twice as good as running!

Moderate runners reduced risks of heart disease by 4.5%, walkers who expended the same amount of energy reduced heart disease risk by 9%!

Getting up from your seat every 30 minutes and moving around for just 5 lowers blood sugar by 20%.

People who walk just 15 minutes after meals see improved blood sugar and better insulin sensitivity for 24 hours!

Remember, improved blood sugar control and insulin sensitivity are not just great for diabetics and those with metabolic syndrome, but for all of us. It's also about appetite control, which is important for long-term weight loss. The number one reported reason for diet failure? Hunger.

From a mechanical perspective, walking is necessary to maintain the health of our organs and their support systems, as we as a species have depended on walking for the health of the pelvic floor, digestion and elimination, being well and strong throughout and after pregnancy, etc.

"But what about my cardio?"

As mentioned above, long-distance, endurance cardio is *not* required for good health. On the contrary, people who run long distances too often can have the similar, shorter lifespans and the higher incidence of heart disease of people who get little to no exercise at all!

The key, according to researchers, is to keep the mileage low and slow when it comes to traditional cardio. A total of 1–2.5 hours of running and the like per week should be fine.

Just an hour? That's pretty easy to fit in to your life, even without expensive cardio machines at home. One or two short jogs or some cycling or skating for fun or transportation, and you're soon in that optimal range.

Resistance training – how strong is strong enough?

Gymrats and weight lifters might think you're weak if you can't lift a barbell that's twice your own weight off of the ground, but in real life, strong enough usually means you're strong enough to carry heavy bags of groceries in from the car, or even just carry your kid up the stairs.

Our ancestors didn't use commercial gyms and weights to get strong enough for life. Your home and your body can often provide enough weight and resistance to build the muscle you need to be healthy and strong enough. Find more information on programs that can take your strength to the next level at eatmovelive52.com.

What happened to flexibility?

Let's define the word "flexible" first. We see people who are amazing at yoga and we're impressed. We see people who are double

---

LIVING IN A WORLD WHERE THINGS WEIGH MORE THAN THREE POUNDS

There are some celebrity trainers who claim a woman should never lift weights over three pounds.

Ridiculous.

When you do one pushup, you're pressing about 60% of your body weight. If you weigh 100 pounds, you're lifting 60 pounds!

When you squat up and down, you're lifting 85% of your weight, or 85 pounds.

When you pick up your child, you're picking up 100% of your child's weight.

Many purses weigh over three pounds. Laptop bags definitely weigh over three pounds! So do most chickens, spiral hams, winter squashes, pot roasts, cast-iron pans, and a bulk bag of broccoli!

Heck, even those tiny little dogs in purses weigh more than three pounds!

Our days are filled with things that weigh well over three pounds, so we might as well be prepared. Start by ignoring advice to put weight limits on your exercises!

---

jointed and we're either wowed or grossed out, depending. Both are flexible.

On the other end of the spectrum, we have the person who's stiff head to toe, who can't squat to the ground to pick up a dropped pen, let alone lift his arms up to the cupboard to grab a bag of nuts.

Flexibility is often defined as the range of motion of your joints or the ability of your joints to move freely, but that doesn't give us the whole picture.

In every movement there are joints that need to be mobile and others that need to be stable; the body is never just flexible or just stable. Flexibility, when increased without strength and control, does not contribute much to overall health and neither does being stiff and stable without having the ability to be mobile in the joints that need to be mobile.

In order to have your joints working at their best, you need them to be mobile first. This is why so many of the exercises we teach you in this book are targeted at working the joints and muscles that are most often stiff and immobile in most of us.

To maintain the newly gained mobility of your joints, you need to get lots of general, natural movement such as hiking, walking, hanging, and the occasional short sprint or strength training workout.

Your fitness goals

Our short-term fitness goals are often things like feeling better and losing weight. For some, it's adding some muscle, too. When looking at longer-term goals, things can seem a little more abstract. What else besides being lean, strong, muscular, and heart healthy is there? Well, there's also bone density, insulin sensitivity, good blood and lymph circulation, plus the byproducts of these things: the ability to live, think, and move – and move well – into old age.

Designing your movement and exercise program doesn't mean going from zero to hero. Even if you're starting from scratch, adding even a little more movement and smart exercise will take you a few steps closer to meeting your health goals.

Like I wrote earlier, exercise, per se, is a supplement to the work most of us aren't doing. If you have a job, sport, or hobby that includes movement, make sure to factor that into your plan. If you're already walking all day long, focus more on the other aspects of exercise, instead.

Your tasks for this chapter:

Now that we've covered the various categories of fitness, exercise, and movement, you get to decide where to start, how much to start with, and how much to add along the way.

Find the step you're at on this list and devote your week to working on it. Then you can work on the next step next week, and so on, until you're a movement hero.

1. **Walk** – The most important and basic type of movement is walking – not power walking, just walking. Unless you're already walking up a storm, take the steps you do now and add to them. Each week, add a little more to each day's steps. Ten thousand steps per day (averaged out over the week) is a good ultimate goal, but that's longer term. This week, just do a little more, and do it every day.

2. **Flexibility and mobility** – Next, start working on mobility. You can do that with the many exercises we outline in this book, which make your office dynamic, get you sitting down

on the ground, or walking with better form. You can find rich corrective exercises to improve your alignment in the resources section at eatmovelive52.com.

3. **Resistance training** – If you already have a good walking habit and are mobilized enough to not feel stiff or achy, start some resistance training to build your strength. Whether you want to train at home or at the gym, with bodyweight or barbells, there is a great program out there for you. Check out the resources at eatmovelive52.com for ideas.

   Resistance training is a higher stress activity, and works best when you limit yourself to between one and three sessions per week.

4. Next, add a little sprinting. Just a few sprints up a hill are all it takes to get the benefits. If hills aren't an option, consider climbing stairs. Hill sprints and stairs are safer than most other forms of sprinting, although sprinting on a stationary bike is a pretty good alternative, too.

5. Still want more? Some moderate traditional "cardio" is fine. If you love running or cycling, keep your total time in this category *under* about two and a half hours per week to keep your heart healthy. Just remember that more isn't always better. Once you've reached this level, it's time to stick with it, and focus more on the other aspects of health, whether it's nutrition, sleep, stress, or relationships.

Where to next?

1. Take Off Your Shoes (p.172)

2. The Best Things Come in NO Packages (p.129)

26 Hanging

by Galina

The missing nutrient for upper body health

On a sunny fall day, I am in Ventura, California, with my friend and mentor, scientist and movement nerd Katy Bowman, and her equally movement passionate husband, Michael. Their kids, at the time one and two, are playing in a sandbox nearby.

Katy, Michael, and I are having a pleasant conversation, during which Katy is hanging by one arm, Michael by two, and I am stretching my legs. This fidgeting party may be a strange sight in the world of adults, but shrink us to the size of five-year-olds, and it would be a common park sight.

What happens between the ages of 5 and 40 that we lose our drive to hang, and ultimately just start "hanging out"? Why do we stop playing and start partying, moving from monkey bars to cocktail bars?

I interviewed Katy, who gave some much needed advice on why and how to start hanging again.

Katy, kids have a drive to hang. They grab on to stuff and swing, play on monkey bars, hang up from furniture, throw their little legs in the air. Where does the drive go when we grow up?

I think we do have that drive to hang even as adults. One of the reasons we may not act on it is we mistake the signals from our body that say "please move in this way." We may be getting the signal, but we interpret it differently. We also learn though upbringing, education, and community to suppress our impulses. Socially, we are inhibited too, you don't see many adults hanging on a structure, so you kind of stay on the side.

Are there cultures around the world or within our culture who hang more?

You'll find lots of kids and adults comfortably hanging in a gymnastics studio. Think of Tim [Restorative Exercise™ teacher extraordinaire]. He hangs all the time, because he used to do gymnastics as a kid, so he has a very living relationship with hanging. He was never separated from the fulfillment of the desire to hang. My dad is also a hanger. He went to a chiropractor when he was 30, and his chiropractor told him to hang every day. He's been doing it ever since. It's like vitamin H.

I know from our training that there are many different ways to hang. If someone is just starting what is a way to introduce hanging?

Before you hang fully you need to get used to placing tension on your arms with your feet still on the ground. Imagine hanging away from a street sign pole – that gentle load would be a great way to slowly start introducing hanging to your shoulders.

I have noticed that when I hang more, my shoulders and grip and back get stronger, but my skin hurts a lot. The skin is limiting my progress. What's that about?

Well, in our modern world we hang on flat and smooth surfaces – like a pull up bar. The smooth surface is not natural, and it's hard to train the skin – it becomes the weakest link. Tree bark is a great strengthener – while the pull up bar will strengthen the muscle, the skin stays weak. Bark provides great stimulus for skin. You can find a tree and start training the skin lightly – different types of bark provide skin cross training. Again, progress slowly.

How do you incorporate hanging throughout the day? With standing, or squatting, or stretching our calves, it seems like there are more opportunities.

Every time I walk through a door I pause to wrap my fingers around the doorjamb. I don't hang, but I do put a load on my body for 10–15 seconds. How many times a day do you walk through a door – 30–40? These are 30–40 hanging moments you wouldn't have otherwise!

You recently posted a cool video of your nephew doing monkey bars. He has a lung condition that improved through hanging, right?

The function of your lungs is in a relationship with the function of the muscles of the thorax. When you don't have optimal thoracic muscular function you limit the mobility of the lungs themselves. In the case of my nephew – his lungs were working in an environment that was already poor. It was partially affected by this poor muscular environment. The inflation of the lungs is brought up by the mobility of the ribs. He was able to strengthen these structures and he was able to get better lung function through the pressure systems that come about by the motion of the ribs.

There is this whole paleo movement out there where it's argued that our ancestors walked a ton. What about hanging, though? Where does it fit? Is hanging a replacement for

something we are not getting, kind of like walking is a replacement for not moving all day for survival?

I would say hanging is something most of us missed as children. Therefore the structures we have were once starved of that movement. We are trying to go back to using these structures in the way they would have been. Around the world there are cultures that have very specific hanging routines for early infants. The bulk of my own kids' hanging does not come from hanging and clambering; it's mostly from holding and climbing onto me. In most cultures children hung on to parents as they were walking and migrating from one place to another. It's a natural movement load that would have come about in a natural setting.

In modern life, we should have the strength to pull ourselves up and into a tree. If you had to forage for your food, there would be many scenarios where climbing or hanging would be a movement nutrient in your daily life.

As Katy's student for the last five years, I've introduced hanging into my daily routine. Anything from gentle hanging on doorjambs, through full swinging on monkey bars. I am not a natural hanger, though.

My lower body has always been way stronger than my upper body. As mentioned in the interview, the skin on my palms is the biggest limiting factor to prolonged hanging. I do, however, enjoy deeper breathing, more shoulder range of motion, zero shoulder pain and stiffness, and much less back pain than ever before. I also have broader shoulders and muscles that show the work!

If you are ready to start hanging, I encourage you to start hanging at the level at which you feel comfortable. Because the load on the shoulders, scapulae, and spine, as well as the wrists and fingers, will be new to you, you will need to give yourself some time to adapt. If you notice you are uncomfortable or too challenged by the hanging that you try, go back a step.

DOORJAMB HANGING

Find a door that you can comfortably hold on to. Wrap the tops of your fingers around the jamb, and slightly bend your elbows. Allow the body to hang down from the door, visualizing the back lengthening. Hold for a few seconds or a minute, being mindful of what you are able to do.

SIDE HANGING

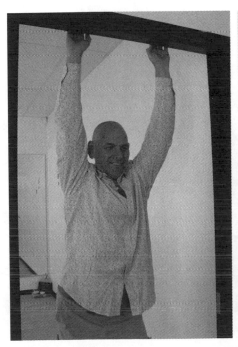 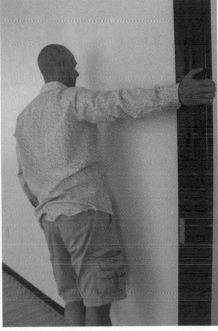

Stand sideways to a parallel or vertical bar. You can also do this with a door. If vertical, your palm will be facing forward and if horizontal, the palm will be facing up. Allow your fingers to grip the bar. Bend your elbow slightly. Allow your body to slightly track away from the bar or door and notice how the shoulder area activates to make your hanging possible.

REVERSE HANG

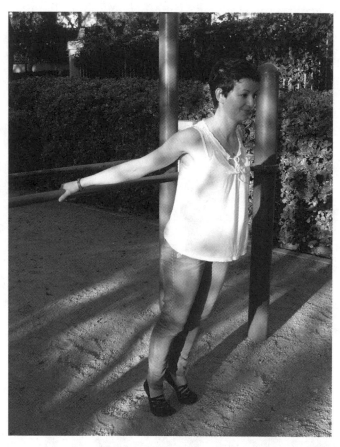

Stand in front of parallel bars. Hold on to the bar with arms behind you and palms facing down. Depending on the tightness in your shoulder area, you may be able to hold the bar with hands closer to shoulder width or wider. Find the position that works for you. Allow the body to drop forward from the shoulders without the hips sagging from the low back down.

TWO-ARM SUPPORTED HANG

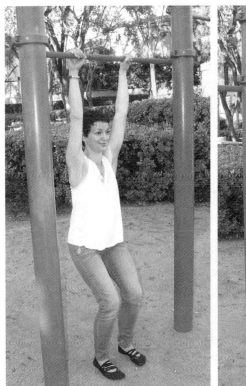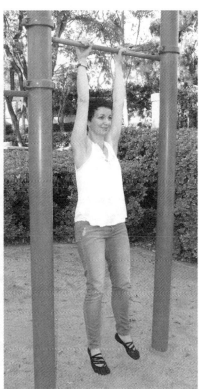

This will only work if you are already able to bring your arms over your head without an arch in your low back, so make sure you know that you are able to do that.

Hold on to a low bar, palms facing away from you. Bend your legs so you are only partially supported by the ground. Allow your body to hang from the scapulae down. Hold for a few seconds. Over time you will be able to hang for 1–2 minutes. Feel free to progress to the unsupported hang when you notice your stamina has increased.

TWO-ARM FREE HANG

Jump or reach up to a high bar, palms facing away from you. Allow your body to hang from the scapulae down. Hold for a few seconds. Over time you will be able to hang for 1–2 minutes.

ONE-ARM SUPPORTED HANG

Hold on to a low bar, palm facing away from you. Bend your legs so you are only partially supported by the ground. Allow your body to hold on by stabilizing the scapula. Hold for a few seconds.

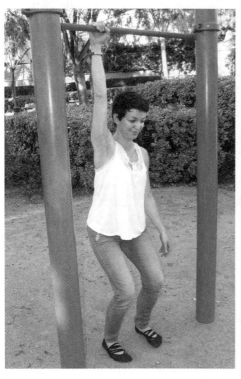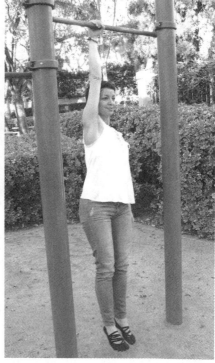

Over time you will be able to hang longer. Feel free to progress to a one-arm free hang when you notice your stamina has increased.

ONE ARM FREE HANG

Jump or reach up to a high bar, palms facing away from you. Let one arm go. Allow your body to hang by stabilizing the scapula. Hold for a few seconds. Over time you will be able to hang longer.

As you start to develop skills in hanging, you can start to introduce more movement, swinging forward or swinging side to side. This will allow you to develop length and strength in the shoulder girdle and enough skill to start playing versus training when you are hanging out at the park.

CHECKING FOR OVERHEAD RANGE OF MOTION

Stand with your back against the wall. Hips and upper back will be touching. Start to lift your arms over your head, elbows straight. You will notice the shoulder blades and shoulder joint move. As your arms come over your head notice what your lower back is doing. If you have to arch it to reach the wall behind you with your arms, then you don't have the necessary shoulder range of motion to hang with your arms over your head yet.

If you find that you don't have sufficient range of motion for a full hang, stick to side-hanging, and practice movements that improve overhead range of motion. After a while, with diligent practice, you may be able to progress to a full hang.

Your tasks for this chapter:

1. Find the appropriate level of hanging that is challenging but also pleasurable for you. Practice multiple times through the day. Notice what feels different in your body – are you more energetic and productive, do you feel more range of motion, can you hold on longer?

2. In your journal, record how often and what kinds of hanging you have been doing. Note as you progress to harder versions over time.

Where to next?

1. Yoga is Not Just for Yogis (p.358)
2. Furniture Minimalism (p.300)

Move Like a Baby

by Galina

27

Happy baby is happy

Your KQ

My teacher Paul enters the room, then gracefully walks to the front of the class and sits down. Legs straight in front of him, palms supported on the floor, spine straight, eyes proud, and silent as a monk, he starts to move.

First the ankles start to move in small circles, and then knees and hips start to roll and bend as he switches one leg over the other. Then with one swift move he is on his back and his legs are scissoring up and down – light as a feather. He rolls over, face down, spine elongated, now his hands are reaching behind his back. From here, up on all fours, he springs into a crawl, first slow, and then fast. Transitions to pushups, down dogs, side jumps, and rolls are smooth and beautiful to watch. At one point, he gets in the "happy baby" position, on his back, legs bent, and grabbing his feet, then he starts to rock left and right, then rolls up to a perfect lotus sit. I am following him, mirroring every movement, sweating like nobody's business.

Ground Force™, a system from Hungary, is a playful combination of natural human movements, which, when strung together, form a logical and exerting workout. You crawl, roll, reach, creep, kneel, lunge, and squat, much like you did before you walked. Funnily enough, you can get a similar workout just by observing and copying a baby or toddler. Good luck keeping up with one of them!

When was the last time you got down on the floor and gracefully got back up? When was the last time you turned over, rolling over to grab a book you left on the other end of the bed, rather than reaching? Have you crawled lately?

In recent years, there has been a steady resurgence of health and fitness systems that challenge us to move like we used to as babies – to spend time on the floor, exploring it with our hands and feet, and moving close to the ground in as many variations and possible combinations of joint angles as we can.

You may be familiar with the notion of IQ, and recently EQ – emotional intelligence, which describes your ability to differentiate between your own emotions and discern other people's emotions. But something like KQ (kinesthetic quotient) or physical intelligence is just emerging. Thomas Myers, author of *Anatomy Trains* and renowned fascia-nado (get it?) points out that if we are to survive the information age in healthy bodies, we must maintain a level of physical intelligence that will help bridge the gap between the movement nutrients our body craves and what we actually end up getting in our movement-deprived reality.

In his words, "Stress is the most ubiquitous disease of the era. Stress is generated by a constant disparity between the 'world as we believe it to be in our inner pictures' and the 'world as reported by our senses'. Given that our bodies are designed and prepared for the Neolithic Era of 70–15,000 years ago, those of us in an urbanized environment are in a constant state of stress."

Most people move in one of three ways: walking, doing some sort of sport or movement art, or doing some sort of rehabilitation exercise. Movers assume that their KQ is high – they can just walk, or just run, or just lift weights, because while they live in their body all day long, it just does what it does naturally – it moves. But take a walk down any street and watch people jogging. Are you seeing the gracefulness of a cheetah, or the worn-down look of exhausted prey? Just yesterday, I was watching a lady run. She was shuffling, mouth breathing, her spine stiff and straight, ankles locked, knees bent. She looked defeated, exhausted, and hurt, like she was at the end of a long run, but she was only just beginning. If that runner had stepped into my office looking for health, I would have created a program designed to increase her kinesthetic intelligence, focusing on touch, rolling, crawling, squatting, pushing, and pulling.

You can easily start to develop a better kinesthetic awareness through your touch sense – using your hands, feet, knees, elbows. Those are the parts of the body that are most richly supplied with nerve endings that give your brain a map of where you are in space, so it can make appropriate decisions when the time comes to walk or run. The body is constantly supplying your brain with rich sensory data coming from the hands, feet, knees, elbows, inner ear, eyes. This is how we rebuild balance and improve movement from the inside out. With basic floor exploration movements you can rekindle the fire of trusting your reflexes – your abs brace as you roll, your neck extends as you look to see where you are heading, your toes find the best angle to push off from.

In my practice I've seen how a program that includes primal human movements not only speeds rehabilitation after injury, but also quickly influences one's movement curiosity, and improves mood, learning, and self-perception.

You start at the beginning, like babies start, with simple movements like rolling and crawling, which help develop the connection between the left and right hemispheres of the brain. This helps both sides of the body coordinate, not only in movement, but also in seeing, hearing, and organ function. The simple act of crawling integrates the neck, shoulders, and hips through the powerful core muscles so you can once again be well wired together.

Smooth, integrated movement patterns are built in our earliest stages of knowing the world through movement. As we begin to move gracefully again, a whole universe of possibilities opens up.

These movements aren't hard, and they are more like fun than they are exercise. As you do them more and more, you might even start to remember how you felt when you did them the first time, as a baby.

BREATHING LEGS UP

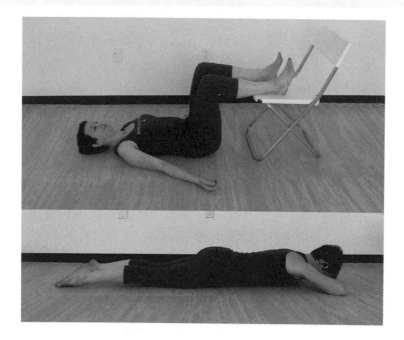

Get on your back with legs up on a chair. Allow your body to settle into the floor. If you need a pillow, get one. Your airway should be straight and free. Inhale through your nose and exhale through your nose. Notice if your belly is lifting, notice if your chest is lifting.

Try to direct the movement in your ribcage, and allow your ribs to expand both sideways and back into the floor. Picture the breath as a 360-degree movement, with ribs free to move out to the side and back into the floor, and your belly gently rising up. Try to quiet the chest as much as you can, and relax the shoulders. Stay in this position as long as you like. Five minutes a day or as a part of your movement practice is best.

BREATHING FACE DOWN

Tummy time! Start by lying face down with your hands under your forehead. Straighten your legs and allow your body to settle. Breathe into your lower ribcage and low back and notice how the front of your body presses against the ground. Notice how the sides of your

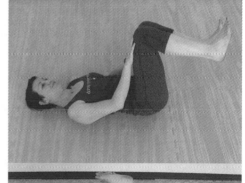

waist expand. Notice how the lower back lifts. Exhale and see how your body sinks into the floor. We call this "crocodile breath" and it's a basic way to get your body breathing before moving toward a crawl. Five minutes a day or as a part of your movement practice is best.

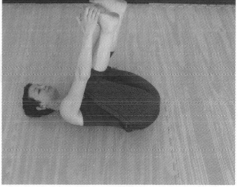

SOFT ROLL

On your back, bring your knees up so your upper legs are vertical. Place hands on your thighs. Gently rock left and right, as far as you are comfortable. Find a rhythm that works for you, and keep to it. Practice several repetitions or till you feel you have gotten the hang of it.

HAPPY BABY ROLL

Get happy by bringing your legs closer to your body and grasping the outside of your feet with your hands. Allow your body to rock left and right. After some practice, you will be able to make it to the floor and back up. Practice for a while, until you feel that it's coming more naturally to you.

X LIFTS

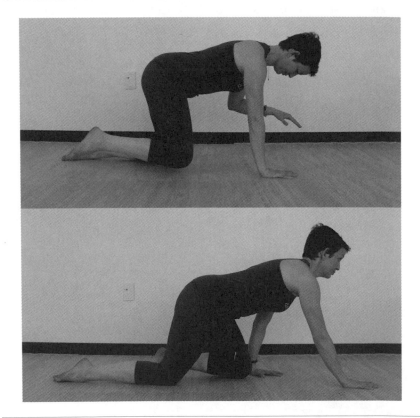

Get on all fours, with your spine and pelvis in their neutral position. You should be relaxed and comfortable. Lift one hand and opposite knee off the floor, then bring them back down. Switch sides. Do this for a minute or so, or until you feel that you have control of the movements and you can feel your body pleasantly connected head to toe.

CRAWLING FORWARD AND BACK

From quadruped, start to move forward, with your hand stepping forward and opposite knee following. Creep forward and back as long as you find it enjoyable. I usually take 4–5 steps forward and 4–5 back. Try going in different directions as well, exploring your environment through this forgotten movement.

How was that?

You may notice, as you practice one or more of these basic exercises, that your mood elevates, your energy increases, and you become more open and relaxed. You can do these on your breaks, as preparation for physical activity, or as a movement practice of their own.

You may want to explore more of the systems that teach developmental patterns of movement. MovNat™ and Ground Force™ are two of the systems that are easily accessible and have many providers that you can locate through their respective websites. For books on the subject, we love *Original Strength* by Tim Anderson and *Smart Moves* by Carla Hannaford.

Your tasks for this chapter:

1. **Move** – Try one or more of the basic floor exercises above, daily, for at least 5 minutes. Notice how you feel, your energy levels, and mood. Like it? Let us know by contacting us at eatmovelive52.com.

2. **Observe** – Watch some toddlers move. Notice how they transition from one movement to another. Try mirroring a toddler for five minutes at a time. For example, when the toddler squats, squat right down with them and spend as much time in that position as they do, then stand back up when they do. Crawling? Rolling? Waving their arms in the air? Join in! When you have a few minutes, head over to our resources page at eatmovelive52.com to watch a fun video of toddlers teaching adult dance classes!

Where to next?

1. Squat Your Way to Health (p.239)
2. Sharpen Your Vision (p.316)

28 Redefine Your Core

The longing for flat abs meets the need for function

T he cult of a flat belly has taken over magazine stands, TV
screens, book covers, and billboards. From "Get six pack abs"
to "Flatten your belly forever," bright pop-ups tell us that there is
a "right" way for the belly to look and that we should probably do
something about the pooch we have where we should have a wash-
board stomach. But the way body parts like our abs look tells us very
little about the way they are functioning.

Somehow over the history of abs we became convinced that the
tighter and flatter the stomach is the better it would work. But
when it comes to the core, that couldn't be farther from the truth.
I propose that you look at your core differently, dare to redefine it,
and start to develop a healthier, more compassionate relationship
with the very structures that house your innermost being – physical
and mental.

When I meet with clients, "the core" is often high on their list of
priorities. They tend to fall into two broad categories: those wanting
a strong core to counteract their sore backs, and those wanting flat
abs to look good. Sometimes a person may want it all – the core
strength to support the back and the flat abs to look good. To most
of them, this seems so simple, but the body is more complicated than
that.

It's important to understand how the body functions as a whole,
rather than looking at individual parts or areas of the body,

MOVEMENT AND EXERCISE   215 otherwise it's easy to oversimplify the approach to returning it to its full capacity. When back pain and injury occur, it's usually the result of faulty movement habits, which have taken decades to develop.

Think of everything you do, from how you get in and out of your car, to how you carry your kid's or groceries, how you squat and do pullups, the position you sleep in, how you stoop over your counter to cut veggies, the way you walk, old injuries and falls. All of these and more contribute to unfavorable movement patterns and pain syndromes.

The traditional advice for addressing back issues has been: Develop a strong core. However, doing isolated exercises for the core muscles will rarely, if ever, give lasting relief, because it does not address how people move when they aren't exercising. Are there people with strong midsections who still function poorly? You bet. Plenty of athletes I work with have very strong-looking cores, can crunch 'til the cows come home, yet fail very basic muscle tests.

Strength isn't everything when it comes to the core. There is an appropriate amount for each muscle, and our body does a pretty good job of activating those muscles necessary to control full body movement, but only when we work our muscle groups as a whole, not in isolation. If we choose to overly work, tense, or brace a certain part of the body, as is common wisdom with training the core, then we deprive our body of the natural ability to fire the right core muscles when it needs them the most. You can be great at an isolated exercise, yet your muscles may still fail to support your back when you need it the most.

On the other hand, a great-looking core doesn't actually require strength. We all have abs under there. In most of us, they are just covered up, and no amount of ab exercise will reveal them if that's the case. If you're worried that you can't look good without doing tons of abdominal work, that very stress could actually be causing your six-pack problems. High stress is correlated with higher levels of visceral fat, likely from increased levels of cortisol. Visceral fat surrounds the internal organs, adds to intra-abdominal pressure, and pushes your belly out, all while disrupting metabolism.

Lowering your stress

If you want to look better in jeans and have a healthier core, you will benefit most from exercises involving relaxation, breathing re-education, losing body fat, and a diet of real food. Adding whole-body activities such as walking or intense hiking will help with your overall energy expenditure, and help you shed pounds without creating extra unnecessary stress to your already stressed system.

Despite what the media shows us, most normal people do not naturally have flat stomachs. The torso is where breathing, digestion, circulation, and elimination occur, and guess what? Those activities need plenty of space. A small, flat belly (especially one that's too tense and tight) can mean trouble!

Try this: Relax your belly, like Buddha. Don't worry about how it looks right now – you can flatten it back when you are done with this exercise. Now take a deep breath, then exhale. Notice how you feel. Now suck your belly in, tighten your abs (like you are going to take a blow to the stomach) – hold this position and inhale. Notice the difference? You simply cannot use your full lung capacity when you're sucking in your belly. Unfortunately, in my practice, I have yet to see a client whose abdominal area is relaxed, much less relaxed enough to function properly. Fed by media and popular health culture, we are all subconsciously holding it in – for fear of looking out of shape, or maybe for fear of our spines malfunctioning on us.

On the other hand, animals do it right. They still rely on instinct, not messages from the media and modern culture. If you have a pet, the next time you see them awake from a nap, notice their reflexive movement – they wake up, stretch, then they start to walk slowly and carefully, observing their environment. They are exploring it for threats, food, and fun. No cat or dog pre-contracts their muscles to look good. Yet, as soon as they are up and going, the muscles in their belly area tense just the right amount to support their quadruped bodies. Why should humans be any different? We're animals, too!

Holding our muscles in, bracing, tensing, and trying to support the back with the abs is not only unnecessary, but potentially harmful. It can get in the way of keeping or creating the reactive core that we want to support and protect our spines when needed. Are six-pack abs really worth all that?

So what do you do?

Assess your belly-holding habits. This is especially important if you have constipation, a history of hernias, prolapse, bladder pressure, prostatitis, diastasis, hemorrhoids, gas pains, or acid reflux. All of those are symptoms of inappropriate core pressure.

Go to a mirror, look at your belly: do you see any lines forming around the muscles, any areas that are more pulled in than others? Can you breathe and feel the belly expand slightly forward, then go back toward your spine? Can you stop holding it in? Can you allow those sharp lines to soften and fill in?

"But it's hanging out now!"

Yes, it is. So was mine. It takes about a month for your natural muscle tone to come back. Remember, holding your midsection in all that time has prevented your reflexes from working, so it will take some time to retrain the muscles. In addition to wearing more loose-fitting clothing, try to walk as much as possible. The more you walk, the faster your muscle tone will return to normal.

ASSESS YOUR ALIGNMENT

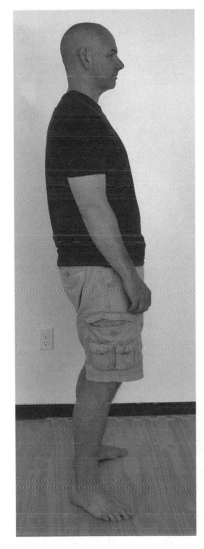 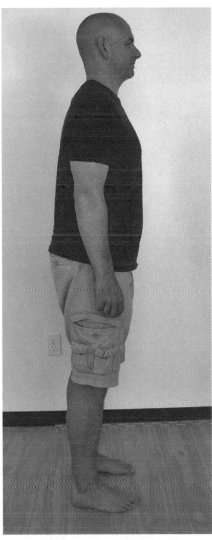

Look at yourself from the side. Is your ribcage directly over your pelvis or do you tend to hold it up farther? We call this rib thrusting or rib shearing, and when the ribs are in front of the pelvis, the body has a really hard time "finding" the appropriate amount of tension for the abdominal muscles. Think of muscle length this way: If a muscle is too long or too short, then activating it at the appropriate time becomes more challenging. Think of Google Maps not giving you a route exactly when you need to go somewhere! Frustrating! When your abdominal muscles are not properly firing to support the body, then the low back muscles often tend to overcompensate and create discomfort and pain. Over a few days, notice if you tend to hold your ribcage in front of your pelvis. If so, gently drop and return the ribs back so they are stacked over your pelvis.

Try reflexive movement

QUADRUPED RELAXATION WITH CRAWL

Get on all fours with your hands under your shoulders and knees under your hips. Try to relax your pelvis so that the tailbone is horizontal to the ground. You will have a neutral spine with a normal S curve and no extra tension. Allow your abdomen to relax.

Now that you have allowed your abs to relax, open yourself to observing what your body does when you start moving.

Crawl a few steps forward, hand first, then opposite knee. Notice what your abs did? Did you see your core musculature respond to your movement? How cool is that? Just the fact that you moved your legs was enough to activate the abs appropriately – no more or less than necessary for this amount of effort.

Now from the quadruped position, lift your knees an inch off the floor. Did you notice your abs fire again? Slowly crawl forward a few steps, then back. Did your abs tense more? Since you are putting

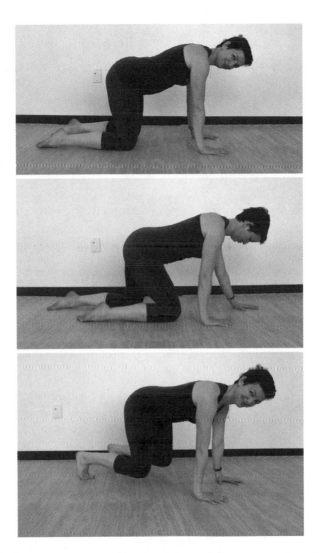

more challenge on your spine in this position, your abs will activate more, without you telling them so. They did it on their own.

As a result of relaxing your belly, realigning your ribcage and pelvis, and introducing reflexive movement, you can expect your core to feel naturally more toned, stress levels to drop, elimination and digestion to become easier, and generally to enjoy a better quality of life. Learning to trust that your body will make the appropriate adjustments when necessary is key to teaching yourself how to have a strong core again. Trust me, nature works better than the man-made idea of what makes for good abs and a strong core.

Your tasks for this chapter:

1. Relax your belly as often as possible. You can do that standing, sitting, lying on your side.

2. Avoid lifting your ribcage up, creating rib shear or a rib thrust.

3. Try getting on all fours and relaxing the belly a couple of times a day. Crawl forward and back for a minute each time and try to get a sense of how your abs activate reflexively.

4. Walk as often as you can. While you're at it, notice how your abs activate during your walks.

Where to next?

1. Eat Yourself Straight (p.72)
2. Slow Down Your Meals (p.22)

29

Bulletproof Your Low Back   by Galina

Bending, lifting, twisting, done right for your low back

My first low back pain was at 11 years old. My parents took me to an orthopedic doctor who twisted and lifted and prodded and poked at me, and then said everything was okay. I was sent home with an exercise routine that I did not do, because it was incredibly painful to even attempt.

I was a classical ballerina at the time, logging hours of dance prep, pointe, and rehearsals for performances each day. When I wasn't dancing I was in school, logging hours of sitting in lectures, reading, and cramming for exams.

To the untrained eye, my body looked great – graceful and long, healthy and mobile. Inside it was a painful mess that only felt better when I moved.

This went on for many years, and in a sense was very educational, as it led me down the path to meet many of the brilliant minds of therapeutic movement. I am lucky to have worked with, been worked on, and learned from some of the smartest people in the health community – but it was also two decades of pain.

One of the approaches that helped me early on was strength training – lifting weights. I learned to better recruit some of my weaker muscles and added lean mass, which helped me stabilize my spine and reduce the pain. However, new aches and pains eventually appeared, and then my shoulders, Achilles, and knees were suffering. I looked strong, but a 20-minute walk was all I could do.

More doctors, but all the MRIs came back negative. Each doctor I saw would assure me that I was fine, but of course "fine" is relative. Maybe they really meant normal, or even just typical.

"Health is the ability to follow your dreams." My dream was to move and teach movement, freedom, and health, and my own body was not reflective of my dream.

In 2010 I met Katy Bowman, a biomechanist who talked about "habits" – what you do the majority of your time with your body – specifically how your body is aligned, or how your joints relate to each other.

Listening to Katy's lectures, it hit me – if I was awake 16 hours a day, spent 1 hour moving with my corrective exercise program, spent 30 minutes massaging my back, yet spent the remaining 14.5 hours holding my body in a position that negatively affected my spine, I had been spinning my wheels. Replacing the habits that weren't serving me with habits that would was my next goal.

I set off to tap into the unconscious, uncover habits that did not serve me anymore, and create new, better ways of moving. I realized this was a much larger and more interesting task than just taking some corrective exercise "supplements." This was the movement equivalent of a "real food" diet.

Over the next six months I became more and more free to move, open to walk, and express myself without limitations. I was able to complete a trip to the mall without pain, I took hikes with heavier backpacks, and started to see that changing habits was way more powerful than managing the pain through supplement approaches.

Clients often ask me why their doctors or therapists do not educate them on habits, and my answer is always the same – changing a habit takes time and effort and comes from the inside out, and only a few dedicated and passionate people will do it. Health specialists focus on providing relief in a way that people are willing to receive it. Lying on a massage table, receiving manual therapy, or popping a new pill takes much less effort than living in your body 24/7 and being responsible for how you stand or walk. We are creatures of convenience, and we do the easy thing. Doctors, if they believed their patients would do the work involved, would probably teach good habits more, and prescribe pills less.

Below, I offer you a few simple ways to integrate a part of my personal practice that allowed me to free my spine for better movement.

Let's start to reacquaint you with your body. The more you feel your spine, the more you understand your spine, the better chance you have of being able to recruit the correct muscles when it's time to lift, twist, chop, punch, run, skip, or sprint. We will start with gentle movements, and over time you will be able to transfer the freedom of movement in your practice to your daily tasks and habits.

SLOW FLEXION

My teacher Michael Curran jokes that it's really hard to move slowly into an injury. Most of us who have been fed corrective exercise for back discomfort or pain tend to hold the spine extremely stiff in order to protect ourselves from movement patterns that we perceive as potentially injurious. Restoring range of motion in the spine and ensuring that each segment can move relative to the other segments is a powerful tool for better movement.

Start by standing with your feet at hip width, toes pointing straight ahead. Drop your chin down toward your chest and transfer weight into the heels. Start to slowly flex the spine, vertebra by vertebra, rolling yourself down toward the floor, visualizing rolling your body forward into relaxation. Direct your attention to the muscles that are holding the spine in extension or tension. Breathe continuously

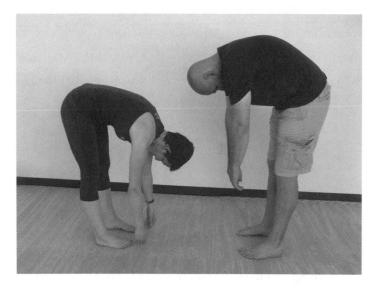

into the spine, allowing each exhalation to relax you forward. If you find a sticky spot, where lots of discomfort occurs or heat is released, back up, inhale, then exhale again to relax it forward. Avoid creating momentum, pulling yourself down with your hands, or adding weight to the movement in any way. Gravity itself will allow you to melt forward. Take about two minutes to come down, head first, tailbone last. Then reverse the movement by using your tailbone to start extending back up, rolling up vertebra by vertebra. Once standing, take a few breaths and walk around a little bit. Then add an extra set.

PRACTICE LIFTING SOMETHING HEAVY

In front of a mirror, stand sideways and make sure that your pelvis is over the ankles, and your ribcage is stacked over the pelvis – this gives you a stable base to use your core and hip muscles to support the back while lifting. If you look at your spine, it has a gentle inward curve in your neck, a small outward curve in the upper back, and a gentle lower back curve. Keep those curves constant as you move.

Straighten your arms down toward the floor and start to sit back into the hips, aiming your tailbone back behind you, while maintaining a neutral spine. Stand back up, only hinging from the hips and keeping the spine stable.

Try this a few times without any weight, then you can try it with objects of varying shapes and weights. A dumbbell or kettlebell lying around your home or gym can make it more convenient, or use a box or laundry basket to practice.

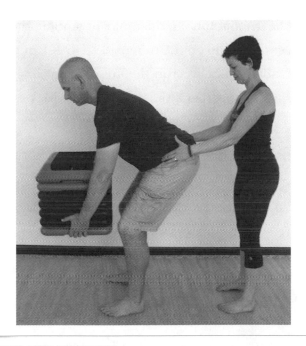

SEATED TWIST

Find a comfortable cushion to sit on. With legs bent, position the pelvis in neutral, so you have a natural neutral low back curve. Relax your ribcage so that your sternum is in a plane vertical to the floor. Start to gently twist to one side, using the muscles on the front

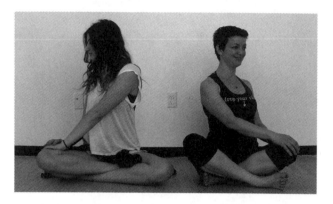

of the torso. Notice if your back is used to recruiting the low back muscles – think of relaxing those before you start to rotate. Slowly rotate to one side without forcing the range of motion, then slowly come back to center and do on the other side. Do 4–5 of these on each side. The more you can recruit the muscles in your abdominal area without overstraining them, the more the low back can relax.

PSOAS RELEASE ON BLOCK

This is like a party for the lower back structures – the deep core muscles that run from the low back to the front of the leg, as well as the musculature between the back of the pelvis and the ribcage. Lie on your back with your knees bent and feet on the floor at hip width. Place your pelvis on a rolled up blanket or yoga block – the pubic bone will be higher than the ASIS bones (the two protruding bones

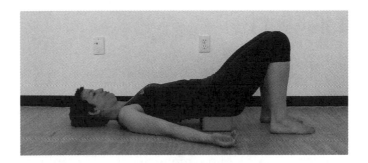

on the front of the pelvis). Let your sacrum be supported, yet let the lumbar spine relax toward the floor. Visualize your lumbar area relaxing into the floor, and tension leaving the spine. Notice that the low back muscles are working because you have been asking them to do so, and let go of that instruction – notice what happens when you do that. This is an excellent relaxation done at the end of your movement practice or daily to get in touch with the habits of tensing your spine.

Your tasks for this chapter:

1. Start noticing when you tense and curl your spine to look straight, position yourself for "good" posture, lift an object, or twist.

2. Start to bring the exercises from this session into your daily movement practice. Notice how one week of doing these daily feels on your back.

3. Head over to the resources section at eatmovelive52.com to see video demonstrations of these movements

Where to next?

1. Detox Your Pantry (p.44)
2. Walking Like Nature Intended (p.154)

30

Roll with It

by Galina

Self-massage for everyone

Have you ever gone to a massage and come out thinking, "Wow, I didn't even know I was that tight there" or "I can breathe so much better!"? Those moments of enlightenment are glimpses into what's possible for most of us – to be able to recognize where in our bodies we store tension and resolve it before it's wreaked havoc on our systems.

I joke with my colleagues that I deal with Mac, iPad, and couch injuries more than I deal with actual falls, breaks, and sprains. Probably 90% of the people I see have a condition related to some repetitive habit or body position that has led to poor tissue quality. A muscle is too tight or unyielding, muscles have stuck together through fascial adhesions, and the flow of life – blood, lymph, electricity – has been interrupted. The area becomes achy and restricted, and movement is compromised.

In a utopian world, every human being would automatically have a massage therapist (and a personal chef and a maid), but that's not reality. If only there was a way to get many of the benefits of massage without going out and spending $100 every time. Well, there is, and it's called self-myofascial release, or SMR. You might have even unknowingly played around with SMR at the gym or yoga studio. Remember that foam roller that hurt so good? That was one type of self-myofascial release.

Over the past few years, SMR has become more and more widespread, with fancy tools, books, education products, and classes available. "Self" refers to, you guessed it, doing it yourself. "Myo" refers to muscles, and "fascial" refers to the fibrous sheath of connective tissue that covers and connects the muscles and organs throughout the body. Fascia is complex, and scientists are still discovering all of its qualities.

According to the *Journal of Bodywork and Movement Therapies*, "fascia is the soft tissue component of the connective tissue system that both penetrates and surrounds muscles, bones, organs, nerves, blood vessels and other structures and extends from head to toe, from front to back, and from surface to deep in an uninterrupted, three-dimensional web."

Picture an orange. On the outside you have the peel. Once you take that off you reveal the individual sections – the carpals – each wrapped in its individual translucent sheath. Opening each sheath, you reveal the individual cells, or juice follicles, each wrapped in its own magically thin membrane. Notice how these structures are all connected – the follicles, the carpals, the pith, and the peel. There is a structure on the surface, but also connecting them, even if very gently, like a complex and wiry 3D web.

The human body is like an orange, only trillions of times richer and more complex in its networks. When we are touched during a massage or we apply pressure on the skin, muscles, and connective tissue, that complex 3D web responds. Through the stimulation of receptors, the muscles relax, fascia slides again, and the flow of electricity, blood, and lymph is restored. When various receptors are stimulated, the brain can better know where you are through a sense of spacial awareness and can make better calculations about creating efficient movement.

With SMR you apply pressure through the use of different tools. You might have tried that foam roller, but there are also balls, sticks, knobs, and other implements at gyms and physical therapist offices. If you already own some of these, then great! These are the tools that will help you tend to the health of your tissues and help you feel better and move with fewer glitches.

My students report many benefits from SMR – better ability to move their hips, shoulders, and spine through a greater range of motion, less discomfort when doing certain exercises or daily activities. They also notice improved balance, strength, and coordination, and a readiness to move where there was caution and fear before. This is both a result of better spacial awareness and better tissue quality.

SMR allows you to target specific areas and smaller tissues, the body's nooks and crannies that are hard to clean up with stretching alone. Some muscles are hard to target with a stretch because of all those pesky other muscles connected to the troubled spot. With SMR you can apply self-release techniques to just one muscle or even a part of a muscle. You can use a ball to focus on just one area of the quadriceps, for instance. Because you can discover the exact spot that feels relief, each session becomes an opportunity for self-evaluation and self-discovery.

Oftentimes, the first encounter with a foam roller on your quads feels like you are rolling over a string of walnuts or coconuts – there are bands and balls of hard tissue that the tool skips over. Those are probably the parts that can benefit most from self-myofascial release's pressure and relaxation. After a few weeks of work, you should notice that those tissues have smoothed out, and you can roll over that area more easily, and without the bumps and tender spots you experienced earlier.

Some degree of discomfort in the areas needing more tender

loving care is typical; as the tissue starts to yield, you will have a more pleasurable experience. More pliable muscles not only feel better and have better flow of nutrients, electricity, and lymph, but also respond better to the input from your brain, so when you move, your movement is smooth and graceful.

SMR using a foam roller, balls, or sticks is an effective, affordable, and accessible way to improve tissue quality at home. Even if you get a massage once every couple of weeks, you can fill in the gaps between massages with your own work.

Are you ready to start?

There are multiple tools to choose from, but the basics you need are a foam roller, a tennis ball, and a massage stick.

Foam rollers – Come in different densities, and if you are purchasing in a store you can press into one and see. For beginners, or people with tighter and more sensitive tissues, a softer roller is more appropriate. For the athletic population or people who don't have a lot of sensitivity to touch, a denser foam roller is great.

Sticks – Come in two basic versions – plastic and rubber foam – and both work fantastic. Sticks are used for areas such as calves and hamstrings that are a bit hard to reach with the big rollers. You lie on a roller to use it, but a stick goes in your hands, very much like a rolling pin.

Balls – A softer rubber ball, a tennis ball, or a dedicated massage ball like a Yoga Tune Up ball is a great way to introduce SMR to a smaller area.

Below are some basic techniques to use with a tennis ball, foam roller, and stick, so let's get started.

TENNIS BALL FOR THE FEET

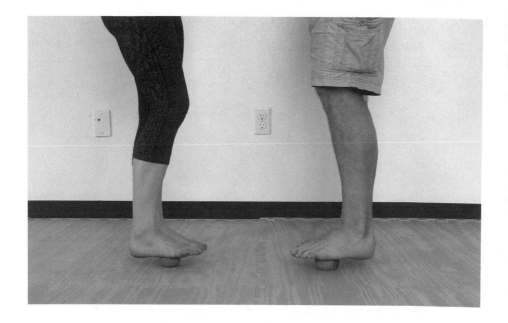

Releasing the feet is important to maintain the health of the lower leg muscles – the plantar fascia that wraps under the foot can get overly stressed from poor shoe choices and lack of movement. Stand with your feet at hip width and place the tennis ball under your foot. Roll back and forth while allowing a significant amount of your bodyweight to be placed over the ball. Do that for 2–3 minutes per foot or as long as you find it enjoyable.

TENNIS BALL FOR THE TRAPS

Stand next to a wall and place a tennis ball behind you. Allow the ball to sink into the bottom of your trapezius muscle. Gently roll up and down and left and right, pressing into the ball; 1–2 minutes should work wonders for tense shoulders and neck.

TENNIS BALL FOR THE CHEST

Stand facing the edge of a wall. Place the tennis ball between your chest and the wall. Picture a line from your mid chest to your collarbone. Roll the ball while applying firm pressure up and down for 1–2 minutes.

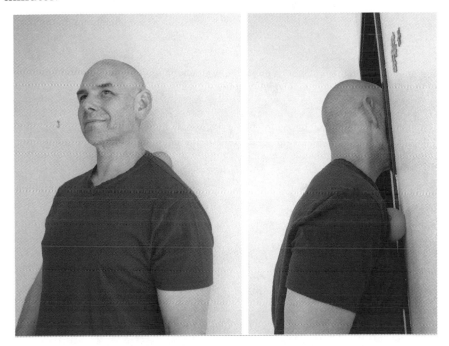

FOAM ROLLER FOR THE BACK

Place the roller at your mid back. Allow your torso to rest on it. Place feet at hip width and shins vertical. Lift your hips off the floor. Hug your chest. Roll back and forth, from mid back to upper back, allowing the upper back to wrap down over the roller.

FOAM ROLLER FOR THE LATS

Turn your body slightly to one side, with the foam roller placed

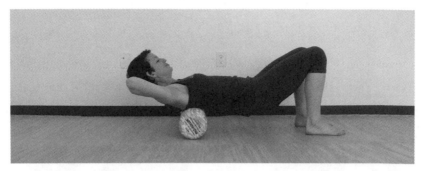

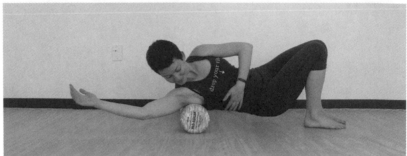

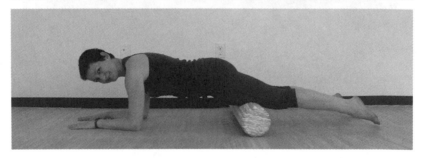

over the lat and teres muscles. Lift your body up and roll back and forth, allowing the body to sink into the roller. Release the area for 1–2 minutes.

FOAM ROLLER FOR THE QUADS

Get in a push-up position, with your elbows on the floor and the roller across your quads. Walk yourself forward and back to roll the muscular tissue of your quads. If you notice certain areas hold more tension, focus on those areas and move with slower and shorter strokes. Release the area for 1–2 minutes.

You can choose to take one leg off the roller and increase the pressure over the other leg. You can also angle your body to the side to release more of the lateral aspects of the quad.

There are companies such as tptherapy.com, yogatuneup.com, and meltmethod.com who provide full kits of rollers, books, and education for those who want to advance in the art of SMR. Not into playing all by yourself? You can find teachers in your area certified to teach those systems, whether in personal sessions or in workshops. A full list of resources for products and courses is available at eatmovelive52.com. We've also provided useful videos for you with more ways to roll with balls, sticks, and foam rollers.

Your tasks for this chapter:

1. If you've never tried SMR, start with a tennis ball massage for your feet. Spend 5 minutes a day and notice how your body changes.

2. For the advanced, try some new exercises. Head over to our website and check out the videos in the resources section. You will learn how to get deeper into your calves, quads, and adductors. Challenge yourself for just 5 minutes a day and notice the difference in your quality of movement!

3. If you like what SMR offers, keep a daily rolling session in your schedule for at least a month. The longer you have been neglecting your tissue health, the longer it will take to restore it. Use the tools to warm up for workouts and hikes, and to recover after a long day.

4. For the office ninja, keeping a tennis ball at your desk and using it to roll out the chest and trapezius muscles can be a lifesaver. Don't forget your feet! Dedicate 5 minutes a day, and let us know how you feel (eatmovelive52.com).

Where to next?

1. Finding Your Fitness Path (p.186)
2. Quiet Time (p.268)

31 Squat Your Way to Health

by Galina

Hey, that floor was made for sitting!

D o you have a toilet?"

"Yes!" The Indian man points Karl at the door and ushers him inside.

"What do I do?" asks Karl, confused and confined within a tiny space that is all walls and door, except for a hole in the middle of the floor.

"Turn around, turn around, face me, and now sit!" instructs his host, gesturing at the hole in the ground.

"What? I can't do that!" says Karl.

"Yes, you can, just sit down, it's better!" insists the Indian man.

"Do you understand how hard this is for me? My insides aren't used to this. Just this morning I came from London. I was sitting ON a toilet, with a NEWSPAPER!" Karl's eyes are wide open in despair.

"But all Indian men use this. It's better!"

"How can this be better? I don't get it!"

"It's better!" insists the Indian man with a smile.

"I hope I don't have to go," says Karl.

This scene is from the brilliant documentary series *An Idiot Abroad* in which Karl, a bland English bloke, is sent off to experience the wonders of the world. He sees poverty, overpopulation, chaos, and dirty streets, but nothing shocks him like the prospect of squatting to poop.

How far have we really strayed from what was once a natural human movement? How far have we strayed from what was natural to us as toddlers? How much has our environment of chairs, cars, cushions, and toilets really changed not only our attitudes, but also our physical ability to get down to the floor, squat to a toilet, or bend over to pick up a dropped pen?

What's in a squat?

The "resting squat" is a well-known concept to most people familiar with fitness and gym culture. This is the type of squat that practically puts your butt on the floor, or "ass to grass." It's a full squat, where you are able to rest in the bottom position, enjoying the full relaxation of torso over upper legs, pelvis opening toward the floor, giving your low back a much deserved break.

Resting? In a squat position? You've got to be kidding me!

You've probably seen a good squat in pictures; cultures all over the world spend significant parts of their days in a squat. It's what my friend Sandy calls the "kimchi squat," since that's how her Korean ancestors positioned themselves to make their famous fermented food.

In Eastern Europe you will often see people resting in the full squat position, and since the squatting toilet is still alive and well in my homeland of Bulgaria, most of us Eastern Europeans maintain a good squatting habit until old age.

Sure, in a chair, sofa, and toilet-oriented culture like ours, the idea of squatting to rest is ridiculous, but around the world, it's a perfectly legitimate position for a coffee break, a game of cards, cooking, or even having lunch. Since the idea of resting in a squat is so foreign to many of us, let's look at some of its other purposes.

A squat is a great way to get down to the floor or a chair for sitting. It's also a great way to get back up again. Squatting comes in handy when you want to do something on or near the ground, like playing with toddlers, gardening without kneeling in mud, or even scrubbing the carpet. It's also the position our ancestors urgently dropped into to relieve themselves until the seated toilet came into existence in the 16th century. Giving birth? That, too, used to be done in a squat.

Yes, the squat is a natural human movement, one that is important when you want to live a full life in a healthy human body.

When we squat, we start by shifting the center of gravity back. Then the ankle joint, hip joints, and spine coordinate their movements to allow a gentle descent toward the floor. The muscles of the trunk and hips work hard to decelerate us, gently, at the bottom. To get back up, the torso muscles and hips generate force to reverse our direction and bring us back to standing. This squatting action, done well, requires mobility of the ankles and hips, and stability of the trunk or core, as well as good breathing mechanics, but our modern lives have robbed us. We've lost ankle mobility by wearing high heels and stiff shoes, and by walking on hard, city sidewalks instead of more natural, varied surfaces. Our hip mobility is shot from a lifetime of sitting, and our torsos are often weakened from a general lack of physical activity, not to mention poor digestion.

When it's time for you, like Karl, to squat down in a foreign bathroom, will your body be there to support you?

Squats are a "use it or lose it" ability – the less you squat and the more you sit, the harder it is on your knees and hips to squat. The more difficult it is to squat, the less likely you are to squat. Whenever you're not squatting, you're actually becoming a worse squatter, minute by minute. That is true of any skill that you rarely work on, and something that involves the coordination between multiple complex joints is easy to lose if not practiced. Your tissues are constantly adapting, as well. If you don't squat, then there is no need to maintain the software and hardware required to do so.

As a personal trainer I have worked with a variety of testing and screening tools to determine what movement skills a person needs to master. One of the first skills we test is their ability to squat. Of the thousands I've watched and tested, almost as many have failed to squat well. In fact, even many of the professional athletes that I've tested have failed to execute a full range, pain-free squat.

Your ability to squat is a direct measure of the many choices you have when you move, use, and inhabit your environment, be it sitting on the floor to play with your kids or grandkids, picking blueberries, or squatting to do a number 2 in the woods. Your squatability is a predictor of your freedom to move and age gracefully, build and maintain appropriate bone and muscle mass in your lower body, and stay healthy and self-sufficient in later life.

If right about now you are thinking that you should head to the gym and crank out 3 sets of 12 squats with some heavy weight on your back, just hold your horses. Good squatting isn't about doing heavy squats in the gym, nor is it the ability to do 200 bodyweight squats following the latest exercise DVD. Good squatting means variety, with different durations, depths, and widths of squats throughout your day.

In a natural, hunter-gatherer environment, for instance, you might squat to pee, then squat to get some tubers out of the ground, do a one-legged squat down from a rock, squat because you dropped something, and squat to talk to some friends while waiting for lunch to cook. Your squats will all have different foot placements, joint angles, depths, durations, and purposes.

When squatting occurs naturally, squats occur many times

throughout the day, not all in one big squat or hundreds in a row. Just like you spread your food and water intake throughout the day, spread your squats out, too.

Be a squat sneaker

I train my clients to be professional squat sneakers. You can learn, too, and have fun while doing it. Here is how you can sneak more squatting into your life.

Use less furniture – Get down to the floor to sit and watch TV and play games with your family. Even if you're not squatting the whole time, simply avoiding the classic sitting position improves your squat instead of hindering it.

If you've already read Roland's chapter on furniture minimalism and going couch-less, then this is just a reminder. If not, then you have a fun chapter to look forward to.

Choose to squat – Whenever you can choose the squat over another movement, choose the squat. Whether it's cleaning the floor, gardening, picking up a pen, or organizing papers, try to do it by squatting. I purposefully squat to organize my messy desk papers and bills, or to scrub the kitchen floor (great for the shoulders, too!). I am sure you can do it too, and you'll get better at it the more often you do it.

Squat to potty – You go to the toilet daily   might as well do it right! Squatting to go not only saves time but also better positions your internal organs for elimination.

Squatting ensures optimal rectoanal angle (straight down) as well as proper pelvic floor tone (relaxed). The pressure of the legs up against the belly also helps elimination, and you can go in one smooth, quick movement. What a deal!

All these sweet benefits are denied to you if you try to eliminate by sitting on a toilet; the extra time spent sitting, plus the extra pressure you need to generate with your pushing can result in a myriad of digestive tract issues, from diverticulitis, to constipation and hemorrhoids. Sold yet?

In 1924, Dr. William Welles wrote about the toilet in his book *The Culture of the Abdomen*: "It would have been better if the contraption had killed its inventor before he launched it under humanity's buttocks."

The 16th-century seated toilet was not exactly suited to the human physiological settings, and even 100 years ago Dr. Welles was alerting readers to the fact that the toileting posture forced by sitting on the can was very different from the natural elimination posture enabled by squatting.

Today there are special stools available on the market, such as the Squatty Potty, that provide a stable platform for your feet, letting you squat directly over your toilet. We've seen people rig up their own squatting boxes, but don't waste your time. The Squatty Potty is now available on Amazon.com for as low as $24.99. The Squatty Potty provides slip-resistant footing, a stable surface, and angled foot beds to help those with poor ankle mobility squat more easily.

How to squat better

You want it all. Shapely toned legs, healthy bones, squeaky clean digestion and elimination, easy birthing, a strong and healthy pelvic floor and abs, and ultimately, independent living and graceful aging. The squat provides all that, and more.

If you are a naturally good squatter, just keep it up. If you are feeling challenged, we have some tips and techniques. You can't just will yourself into a good squat, after all. You've got to help your body relearn the movement that once came naturally.

Squat Prep Routine

Our squat prep routine includes some simple stretching and some assisted squatting movements that help retrain your body, mind, and nervous system to squat better. Better squatting, done regularly and often, leads to better squatting over time.

Do your squat prep routine daily, if not several times per day. This might sound like a lot, but you're just trying it out for one week for now. If you make significant progress and get into the habit, you'll find it easier and easier, and less intrusive on your life. One day you'll find yourself simply squatting more easily, and then you'll be on your way to a lifetime of good squatting, and all the benefits that go with it!

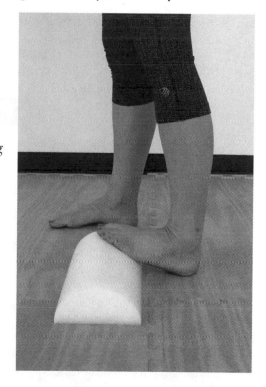

CALF STRETCH

We write about calf stretching quite a bit in this book. That's because there are so many things in life that limit our calf length, and limited calf length affects so many things in life. The shortness and stiffness in calves and ankles is one of the biggest limiters of people's squats.

Grab a towel and roll it up to the thickness of a wine bottle and put it in front of you. Space your feet hip width apart. Step forward and place one foot at the edge of the towel, keeping the foot straight. Walk forward with the other foot until you feel a stretch in the calf of the front foot. Keep the pelvis from rotating and do not bend at the waist! Keep weight in the heel of the stretching leg and both legs straight. You can step forward or back to adjust the amount of stretch. Hold for a minute on each side and repeat several times.

SQUAT ON ALL FOURS

Get on all fours. Position your knees so they are the width of your hip joints and your feet are at the same width. Tuck toes under. Check that your pelvis is not tucked under – it helps to stick your butt back and allow the spine to take its natural S-shaped curve. Slowly sit back, pushing your pelvis back behind you, but minding that you maintain the spinal curves. Sit back only as far as you are comfortable and come back to center. This is the same hip joint mobility drill as doing a squat but minus all the drama of gravity.

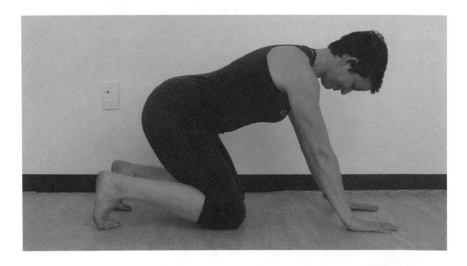

DOORKNOB SQUAT

Hold on to a doorknob so you have some support to hold yourself straight up. Place your feet at hip width with toes pointing straight.

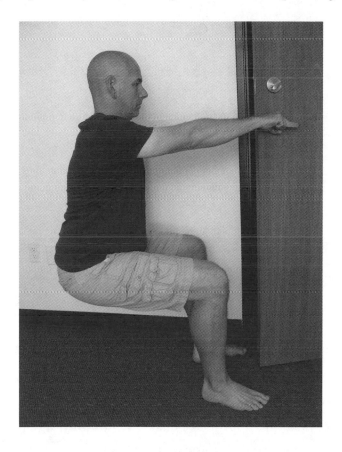

Start to sit back into a squat, maintaining your spinal curves and allowing movement to happen at the hip joints. Make sure your tailbone does not curl under you. Ideally you want to go back down enough so your upper legs are parallel to the floor. Feel your glutes support you down there, push off through your heels, and stand back up.

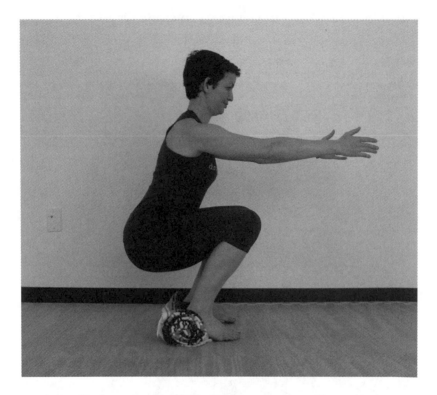

Grab a rolled-up towel or a half-dome foam-roller and place your heels on it. Now slowly drop into a deep squat. Relax and enjoy for as long as you want.

Television time is great for your Squat Prep. But if you're not a TV person, don't start now! Music and podcasts are a wonderful way to pass the time while stretching.

Your tasks for this chapter:

1. **Squat prep**: Do your squat prep routine several times per day, and see how much progress you can make, even in just one week!

2. **Squat more**: Play with and get used to the squatting position. Squat to get down to the floor and back up again, squat to pick up something you dropped, to clean, or to play, even for a few minutes at a time.

3. **Get a Squatty Potty**: There are benefits that come directly from squatting while pooping, such as better digestion, less constipation, easier, more thorough elimination, and fewer bathroom related ailments, such as hemorrhoids.

Where to next?

1. Meditate on This (p.340)
2. Just Look, You Don't Have to Touch (p.142)

32

Let It Go...

by Galina

...and become a stress pattern detective

A herd of impala grazes peacefully in a lush wadi. Suddenly, the wind shifts, carrying with it a new, but familiar scent. The impala sense danger in the air and become instantly tensed to a hair trigger of alertness. They sniff, look, and listen carefully for a few moments, but when nothing appears, the animals return to their grazing, relaxed, yet vigilant.

— Peter Levine, *Waking the Tiger*

Animals have developed fantastic mechanisms to stay safe in nature – camouflage, burrowing, freezing, or in some cases attacking. You may have experienced the mama bear response if your child or a loved one was ever in harm's way. Instincts take over, and suddenly you are acting from a place of pure instinct, submitting to nature's embedded operating system that takes over to ensure survival.

You might have heard of fight or flight, but there's a third option built into us: freeze. In a dangerous situation, you may choose to engage your opponent or run away. When neither is an option, a third action – freeze – is implemented. It doesn't really matter to your physiology which route you go, as the goal is just to make sure that you can survive until the danger has passed. This primitive survival response is installed in your human brain.

As a biological entity we are always responding to the environment – and our bodies are constantly filtering the stimuli from noise, light, computers, calls, thoughts, plans, and turmoil, and choosing whether to fight, flight, or freeze. At the end of a day full of stimuli, unlike the impala from the quote above, we may not return to a state of relaxed vigilance, but remain in a state of tension and discomfort.

I work with the tensest of the tense – people who have endured multiple traumas, deal with anxiety, work high-stress jobs, and manage large families and organizations. Over the years, I've developed an eye for biological tension.

Not making eye contact. Slouching. Mouth breathing. Shoulders high. Neck tense. Talking a mile a minute. Not talking much. Elevated heart rate. Increased blood pressure. Back pain. Neck pain. Thyroid meds. Antidepressants. Muscle relaxants. Incontinence. Pelvic pain. IBS. Allergies. Asthma.

I can see it in their bodies, I can read it in their intake forms, even when they don't spell it out.

The fight-flight-freeze response is supposed to be a short-term survival strategy response, not a long-term interest rate we pay for staying alive. When faced with an attacker, you want your adrenals to be flooding your blood with hormones to kill pain, increase vigilance, give you superhuman powers, and allow you to kick your opponent's butt. When the threat is gone, hormones should start to quiet down, breathing and heart rate will drop. You, dear human, should now be able to keep "living and grazing, relaxed."

In an ideal scenario, we have time to process what happened after a stressor hits us. We will have time to recover from the fight or flight and thaw from the freeze. In nature, the discharge of the powerful hormonal energy of survival can come as trembling, shaking, heat. The arousal will be followed by a deactivation, and a response of peace and physiological, emotional, and mental relaxation.

But what happens when our environment is constantly poking us in the ribs, making our bodies react viscerally with the fight-or-flight response? What happens when it's inappropriate to kick, scream, scratch, or sprint for the conference room door? The instinct is there, you are charged up and ready for action, yet the action never happens.

Your muscles never get to express the energy that is charged within them, so at the end of the day you go home exhausted, with residual muscle tension in one or more places in your body. Over time, that tension can cause pain, discomfort, limited mobility, migraines, pelvic floor and digestive issues, joint pain, and in extreme cases complicate syndromes such as fibromyalgia and other conditions that might be triggered by stress.

The good news is that you don't have to be a slave to the fight-flight-freeze response and you can help your own body discharge the energy built up within your tissues. It takes some practice and some mindful awareness, but it's pleasant and very easy to learn.

This is the very sequence I use to gain control of my stress patterns: self-observation, relaxation, and environment integration.

First, start with self-observation. Tension usually manifests as sensations of constriction, limited blood flow, local stiffness, muscle knots, and dull aches and pain. Sometimes stiffness limits your movement, such as not being able to rotate your head to look behind you, or not being able to straighten your back after sitting.

The biggest areas of tension are shoulders, neck, jaw, brows. Think frowning, clenching teeth, grinding teeth, tearing apart with your teeth, turning your head left and right, lifting the shoulders up toward your ears, punching, and grabbing. Hands, as in making fists, can also exhibit a lot of accumulated tension. Going south, the belly, low back, pelvic floor, butt cheeks, quads, and toes are also on my tension radar when working with clients. Most people accumulate tension in multiple areas.

Females are especially prone to abdominal and pelvic floor tension, because of the pressure to look thin and have flat stomachs, and we are also more likely to suffer from pelvic floor pain and digestive disorders because of the resulting stress and anxiety.

Find your tension

Start standing or sitting, but we'll do our tension detective work from the top down.

Brows – Start by frowning. Notice how your face feels when you frown, then relax into a natural smile and exhale as you let go of the heaviness of the frown. Notice how that feels in comparison. The small muscles that help you frown – the corrugators – can be chronically tense. Allowing them to chill helps the whole body chill out.

Jaw – Place your hands on your cheekbones. Clench your teeth and notice how the firm muscles of the jaw – pterygoids and masseters – pop up in your hands like lollipops, stiff and hard. Now open the bottom jaw – literally, drop your jaw – and sense how they feel when they are relaxed. This is how you want them to feel all the time. If you can learn to keep the teeth gently separated and the tongue on the roof of the mouth, lips closed, this ensures optimal airway position for breathing and minimal jaw tension.

Shoulders – Shrug them up and tense them as much as you can. Don't just do a half-hearted I-don't-know shrug; go for the full crunched up, yucky, uncomfortable squeezing the shoulders up toward the ears. Notice how tension feels. Now exhale and let it go. Allow your shoulders to drop away from the ears, down in relaxation land. How do you like that?

The goal is to notice tension, and you can only become good at noticing what you have experienced, so by practicing tension and relaxation you will get better at finding your patterns.

Fists – That's an easy one. Make a fist, then let it go. A nice variation on this for those of you who handwrite a lot is to squeeze your pen or pencil, then let it go. You want to be able to hold your pen with the least amount of effort, instead of squeezing the life out of it.

Belly tension – It's probably easiest to stand up for this one. Tense your abs as if you are getting ready to take a punch from someone. Hold it like that. Make sure you are still breathing. Now let the belly go. All. The. Way....No, seriously. All. The. Way.

Pelvic floor – Those "down there" muscles may be a little harder to feel than your biceps. In a busy work environment most pelvic floors get overly tight due to delaying going to the bathroom. Just one more email, just one more call. While number 1 or 2 have to wait for you to get your work done, the muscles down there are working overtime. Day after day, that can result in tightening and weakening of the tissues. Pelvic floor tension also increases under mental stress, and millions of men and women suffer from pelvic floor tension–related disorders such as prostatitis for men, or prolapse and painful intercourse for women, without even realizing that their body is overreacting to the stimulation from the environment.

To locate those muscles and become aware of them, squeeze the same muscles you use when you are trying to stop urinating, then let them go. Let them go enough so you feel no tension in that area. You can do the same with your anal muscles, as well as your butt cheeks. Because of the proximity of the large gluteal muscles to the pelvic floor, tensing them to look good in a pair of jeans can wreak havoc on the whole pelvic bowl. So, several times a day, check with that tension and make sure you are as relaxed as possible.

Quadriceps – Here come your Olympic speed skater muscles. Many of us tend to keep the front of the legs tight as we stand. While you are reading this, stand up. Notice where your weight is distributed. Ideally, you should have your pelvis resting over your heels, so a large amount of your weight is placed on the long bones of the leg. Your hamstrings and glutes should be doing some of the work in this position, with only a small amount of effort coming from the quads. Tense up the quads – you will notice the kneecaps come up and in toward the knee joint. Now relax the quads – the kneecaps will descend. This is your no-tension quad mode. How do you like that?

Toes – Last, check what those little piggies are doing. Grasp the floor with your toes, now let them go and relax them. Your toes should be free to move at all times so that when you choose to walk, jump, or lunge, the muscles attached to them can work, instead of doing the work of other muscles up the chain. See, when you have a weak core or hips, the toes will grip the floor for dear life, and then, you guessed it, not be able to do their own work. There are 26 bones, 19 muscles, and over 100 ligaments in the foot. They have a lot of functions to perform on their own. Holding extra stress in the toes can hinder natural performance. To make sure you have not created crazy stress patterns in your toesies, just check with them regularly.

Use the image at the top of the next page to check for tension multiple times a day. You can also print it out and stick it to your computer monitor or fridge as a reminder until you have formed the habit of letting stress go.

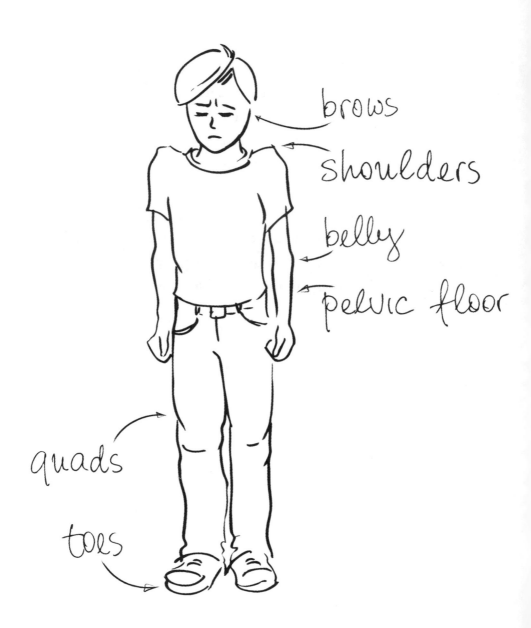

brows

shoulders

belly

pelvic floor

quads

toes

Once you have become quite good at all-day tension release, you may feel much better. I still recommend you dedicate 10–15 minutes a day to do the following relaxation exercise:

THE PSOAS RELEASE EXERCISE

The goal of this relaxation exercise is to ease the tension in your deep core and lumbar area. It also helps you connect with areas that are chronically tense because of mental strain and negative thoughts.

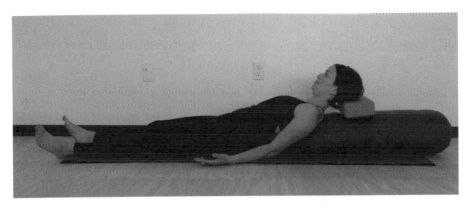

First, fold a large blanket until you have it square to the thickness of a firm pillow. Place it on the ground and grab a small pillow.

Before you go into the release, lie on your back and assess how tense or relaxed your body is. Check your chin position, the shape and contact of your shoulder blades on the floor, how far your spine is from the floor in its different segments, whether the backs of your thighs are relaxed on the floor or lifted off the floor, where your pelvis is and generally how relaxed on the floor or lifted off of the floor you feel.

To set up for the release place your shoulder blades on the folded blanket (or yoga bolster). Place the small pillow or yoga brick under your head so that your chin can drop down and relax. Place your arms at your sides, palms up. From here you can assess the elevation of your ribcage – you can touch your ribs and see how far they are sticking up, out, or to the side. Ideally the ridges of your ribs should be flush with the flesh of your abdominals and not visible at all. Gently breathe in and breathe out, allowing the chest to relax towards the ground and the low back to ease into an imaginary hammock.

Allow yourself to rest in this position for 10–15 minutes. Then move back to the flat floor and check how your spine, pelvis, and lower body feel. Much better, huh?

You can do this anytime, but preferably when you are home and getting ready to wind down. This exercise relaxes you both physically and mentally and can prepare you for a great night's sleep.

Once you have relaxed, you are ready to do environment integration. That is just a fancy way of saying "noticing what's going on around you."

THE NOTICER EXERCISE

You can do this after tension check, psoas release, or anytime you feel a need to get in better touch with your senses. You need something to look at or touch – preferably something you enjoy.

I look out the window. I let my eyes go where they want to go. They go to the tree right outside our kitchen. I explore the leaves – the light green color, the texture, the shape, the way they move in the wind. I feel the motion as if I was outside and this brings a warm smile to my face. I then notice the bark. Some ants are going up and down, carrying building material. Funny little guys.

You can stay present with what you are observing for as long as you like and notice how that shifts your emotional state and your physical sensations.

Your tasks for this chapter:

1. Become a tension detective: Check your tension, and let go of at least one pattern you notice. Jaw clenching? Shoulder scrunching? Let. It. Go.

2. Do the psoas release at least once this week, but more, if possible. You can see a video guiding you how to do it in the resources section at eatmovelive52.com.

3. Do the noticer exercise after you relax a body part or anytime you like to. It will bring peace and awareness to your day.

Where to next?

1. Yoga is Not Just for Yogis (p.358)
2. Now This Sucked (p.367)

Explore Your Breathing
by Galina

33

What if your most natural movement doesn't always come naturally?

Breathing happens tens of thousands of times a day, right under your nose. The average adult breathes between 15,000 and 25,000 times a day. If you did 20,000 squats a day, wouldn't you be concerned about form?

Stress, sedentary lifestyle, restrictive clothing, and forced "correct" posture have made natural human breathing a rare phenomenon to observe. Most of us don't breathe in easily or fully, and exhale just as poorly, never being able to experience a full, deep breathing cycle. Tense necks and upper backs, achy lower backs and immobile shoulders and hips are just some of the manifestations of poor breath mechanics – add digestive distress, stress, anxiety, low energy, and you have yourself a perfect picture of the modern human.

We tend to pay attention to the mechanical aspects of breathing. We take a deep breath to calm down, or exhale fully in yoga class, but most of us don't realize that our skeleton and organ position and alignment can help or hinder the mechanical breathing process. If you position your body well for optimal breathing, the mechanics of breathing will work easily on their own, without you having to force the breath in. The reverse is also true, and ultimately more common in the Western world, with our chairs, cars, and computers. It's a rare thing when our bodies are aligned as nature intended, and our breathing suffers.

The trouble with not paying attention to things that are or should be happening on their own is that we may believe everything is okay, even when it's not. Slowly, our environment shapes our bodies in ways that may hinder optimal breathing, yet it's happening so slowly over time that we don't notice that something is off. To illustrate this better, let's do the following alignment explorations together. You will need a chair or exercise ball.

While exploring these positions, you will find more optimal positions to inhale and exhale, improving your breath, reducing tension and stress.

1. **Head position** – Keep your torso upright. Move your head forward like you are trying to see some fine detail in front of you. Inhale through your nose and exhale through your nose. Take note of how free your breath feels and how much your lungs inflate. Then gently take the head back to rest over the shoulders. Inhale and exhale again and take note of how that felt. Notice how the head position changes your airway and the ability to take in a full effortless breath of air. Does the air just come in, or do you have to suck it in? The less effort,

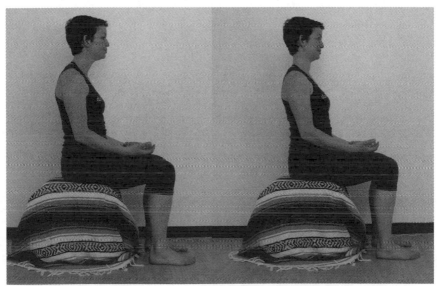

the better. Head position is a common reason for suboptimal breathing and a lot of tension in the neck muscles being used to "suck" the air in.

2. **Tongue position** – Keep your head in the aligned position from the exercise above – with the ear over the shoulder. Place your tongue on the floor of your mouth. Inhale and exhale, taking a few full natural breaths. Take note of the effort it takes to draw in the air and how much and where your torso inflates. Now move your tongue to the roof of your mouth and gently press it and spread it like you are smiling from the inside. Inhale and exhale a couple of times and notice if there's a difference. Believe it or not, this simple change allows the back of the throat to open as the tongue lifts up and away and allows for a larger airway. Oftentimes lack of stability in the jaw provided by this tongue position can lead both to suboptimal breathing and neck tension and discomfort.

3. **Ribcage up** – While sitting with head over the shoulders, lift the ribcage up, like you are standing up really straight, and pull

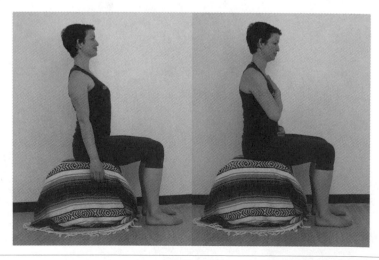

your shoulder blades back like your mom taught you. Take in a deep breath and notice how that affects the direction of the breath and the movement of the lungs and ribcage. Then bring your ribcage down so that the ribcage is vertically stacked over the pelvis. Relax the shoulder blades so that they are at the widest possible position on the sides of your ribcage. Take in another few breaths and notice how much easier it is for your body to breathe when you are not creating extra tension in the system. Chronic pulling of the shoulders back not only limits the body parts that participate in breathing, but also often creates a pattern of low back tension and discomfort.

4. **Pelvis tucked** – Sit with your pelvis tucked, like you are slouched and sitting on your tailbone. Take a few deep breaths in and notice how your body responds. Now align your pelvis sitting forward on the ischial tuberosities with your tailbone behind you and your spine nice and tall. Notice how much space opens between the ribs and the pelvis. Take in a few deep breaths and enjoy.

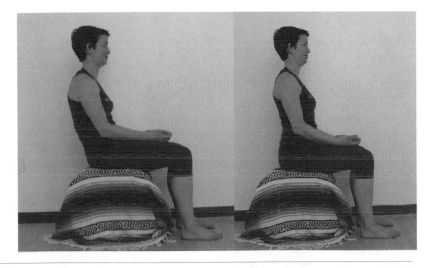

The four key elements above – head and tongue position, ribcage up, and pelvis aligned – are really easy to implement. Together they will ensure that your parts are all positioned for the beautiful and synchronized act that is breathing. Let's try it.

Inhale. As you do, air comes in through your nose, and it's both warmed and sanitized in the process. It reaches deep in your lungs, as the diaphragm contracts down and the ribcage expands. Your pelvic floor also stretches and relaxes. While you exhale, oxygen is being delivered to all cells, and the diaphragm and pelvic floor lift back up. Picture the whole process as a wave going down and then going back up, yet the wave is only as efficient as the position of your body parts.

Signs of suboptimal breathing may be obvious – such as getting tired easily, feeling like you need to take in air forcefully, or holding your breath. They can also be masked as many other conditions. Because the health of all systems depends on a constant and reliable supply of oxygen, many symptoms overlap. You may also experience stress, anxiety, irritability, depression, low back pain, neck and jaw tension, migraines, digestive distress, poor sleep, weight gain, pain and fatigue with exercise, dizziness, chronic fatigue, and a weak immune system.

Whether you are sitting, walking, or resting, make sure you have your head stacked over the shoulders, and your ribcage stacked over the pelvis. If you don't check in with your alignment periodically, a predominantly sedentary modern lifestyle can lead to misalignment and mal-positioning of your head, ribcage, and pelvis in a way that hinders effortless and efficient breathing over time.

Nose breathing vs. mouth breathing

Once you have addressed your optimal alignment for breathing, you want to pay particular attention to nose breathing. Many people breathe though the mouth, and in the process bypass the most basic and beneficial way we are designed to breathe. Breathing is so important (duh!) that nature has provided two ways for us to breathe – through the nose or through the mouth. Consider the nose your primary way to inhale and exhale, and your mouth as your emergency, plan B route. You want to be able to breathe through the mouth if your nose is clogged, or, for example, if a tiger is chasing you and about to get you. However, mouth breathing tends to be shallow, upper chest breathing, and doesn't provide the same benefits as nose breathing.

Nose breathing warms, humidifies, and sanitizes the air, improves circulation, optimizes oxygen and CO_2 levels, slows the breathing rate, and allows lungs to stay pre-inflated for easier and more efficient breathing – thus maximizing lung volume and the ability for the body to extract oxygen. If you are finding that breathing through the nose is hard, you may want to consult an ear, nose, and throat doctor for help.

If you are cleared by the doctor, and don't have a condition that requires medical attention, many people react well to natural nasal sprays such as Xlear or the Neti Stick – they can often help with the environment in the nose by unclogging and minimizing mucus. Another good tool is the Breathe Right nasal strip – placed directly on the nose to open it up for more efficient breathing. Chin-Up Strips are another option to try. They are placed on the chin to help with persistent mouth breathing.

Positioning your body for optimal breath is easy, inexpensive, and has carryover to many areas of life. Many of our clients who transition to nose breathing and follow the basic alignment principles above notice marked reduction in stress, less anxiety, improved sleep duration and quality, more energy and creativity, better digestion, less fatigue during afternoon hours, reduction in chronic pain, and improved overall well-being.

It's time to try for yourself!

Your tasks for this chapter:

1. Try the four alignment exercises from the start of this chapter. Explore and find the most optimal positions for work, rest, and movement.

2. Take nose breathing with you wherever you go. Simply close your mouth and allow your nose to do the work.

3. If you know that you have a breathing challenge, there are many modalities which help with restoring your breathing mechanics, such as PRI, DNS, Buteyko Method, Nutritious Movement™, and Restorative Breathing.

4. Come to our website and try additional exercises that coordinate breath and movement – you can find them at eatmovelive52.com.

Where to next?

1. Meet Your Feet (p.164)
2. Redefine Your Core (p.215)

WORK, HOME, AND LIFESTYLE

34

Quiet Time

Finding silence in a world that will never be quiet again

Insidious noise pollution

I often work from home in the mornings before heading out to see clients. Working from home is not always all it's cracked up to be. Recently, I complained on Facebook about the city's gardeners edging, mowing, and leaf blowing under my window starting as early as 7:15 every Monday. Monday is bad enough, but it wasn't just Monday. On Tuesday, our apartment complex's gardeners do the same thing, still under our windows, but inside the complex rather than along the city streets. That Wednesday, another group of gardeners stopped by to trim the hedges under the window. And on Friday, another group of gardeners came to leaf blow our entire complex free of leaves for the weekend. At least I'm learning the schedule.

Back on Facebook, several people agreed that it was a problem, but a few people suggested that I was being a whiner. One even said, "So sorry for your first-world problems." Is it really a first-world problem that I don't want hours of loud engine noises disrupting four out of my five workdays?

Maybe the real first-world problem is that people feel such a need for carefully manicured plants and grass. The strange desire for streets, sidewalks, and parking lots totally free of leaves is strong enough that we are willing to suffer through hours of noise pollution. I wonder how an old-world village would react if you sent in a gardening crew to loudly blow all the leaves away four times per week.

Noise pollution is a real problem, but it's insidious; we tune it out.

We push it to the back of our minds, but it's there, distracting us at best, making many of us edgy and unproductive, and in the worst cases, contributing to high blood pressure and even cardiovascular disease and mental illness.

The evolution of noise

It's only been a few hundred years since we've been exposed to the levels of noise that we are today. It's only been a few thousand years that we've lived in cities and been exposed to constant, low-level noise. We evolved during quiet times, and we certainly aren't yet biologically used to our loud world. Studies into what noise pollution does to our health show hearing loss, headaches, high blood pressure, speech interference, poor sleep, and lost productivity. And it turns out that people exposed to constant levels of noise, such as airplane engines and street traffic, are admitted to psychiatric hospitals at higher rates than those in quieter neighborhoods.

Types of noise pollution and what we can do about them

No matter the health-related issue, I encourage people to change what they can, control what they can control, and minimize the rest. This is as true for handling your exposure to noise as it is for your diet or exercise regime.

With noise pollution there are three basic aspects to deal with: loud noise, ambient noise, and, strangely, lack of silence.

Loud noise, such as airports, traffic, powered gardening, sirens, industrial noises, power tools, and loud music

When it comes to loud noises, it's important to have good ear protection and reduce the time of exposure. We see airport personnel and gardeners wearing ear protection, but home gardeners and weekend carpenters rarely do. Buy some and use it.

We like our music loud, but constant exposure and competing noise (music and otherwise) slowly build up our tolerance, so we pump up the volume even more.

Protecting your ears and reducing your exposure to loud noises over time should help to reset your sound preferences. In the meantime, try actively listening to your music a little quieter. Use ear buds that block out ambient noise rather than cheaper headphones that need to be cranked up to compete with the outside world.

Ambient noise (coffee houses, chatter, televisions, radios, and background music)

Some of us work better when we are surrounded by ambient noise. My suspicion is that we get used to the lack of silence, and find comfort in constant, if non-specific, noise. Even when alone, the TV talks to us, and many people are comforted by being around people at Starbucks, even when they sit alone and talk to no one. Today, noise can be comforting where silence probably comforted our ancestors.

Many of us have no choice but to deal with ambient noise, often resorting to blasting our own music louder in an attempt to make the outside noises even less specific to us. Yes, you still hear the hiss of the espresso machine, but it's background noise now. When the blender blends, we turn up the volume, and in an attempt to put ambient noise farther into the background, we push ourselves further into Loud Noise territory.

Can you see how these things build on each other?

Lack of silence (headphones on all the time, living in civilization, and never giving yourself a noise break)

Lack of silence? How can something that isn't even a thing be a problem?

We, as a species, developed in *silence* compared to the constant noises that we live in today. We think we need the noise, but we're just used to it, and over time have come to expect it. While avoiding the loud noises and cutting down on constant ambient noise is important, seeking out silence, and the environment where it's found, might be the most beneficial act of all.

Look for silence. The world is never totally quiet, but you know natural silence or quiet when you (don't) hear it. Find opportunities to get quiet as best you can. The *act* of finding your silence has benefits beyond merely not hearing all that noise.

You might have heard of *shinrin-yoku*, a Japanese term meaning "forest bathing." Forest bathing has nothing to do with washing up or being nekkid. In the most general way it means "being in the forest for health purposes," enjoying the peace and quiet, and relaxing. *Shinrin-yoku* works well enough that it's a prescribed stress reduction therapy in Japan and Korea.

Keep in mind 100% nature and 100% quiet are not required. We have a regional park near us, and technically it's surrounded by highways, even though you can't see them. When I go there and find a tree to climb or rock to sit on, I feel the quiet. Yes, I can listen hard and hear the sounds of traffic off in the distance, but the woodpeckers, squirrels, and bubbling streams win this time. For my purposes, my park is quiet.

Your tasks for this chapter:

1. If you work with loud noises, head to the store and buy some ear protection and use it. The type of noise and how often you're exposed will help you choose from among simple ear plugs or those high-tech earmuffs like the guys who gave

Maverick the thumbs up to take off in *Top Gun*.

2. Upgrade your sound. If you're wearing headphones that force you to crank the volume to hear over that guy next to you, it's dangerous to your hearing, and time to shop for better sound. Studies show that people who wear earphones that fully cover the ears actually listen at lower volumes because they don't have to cover up all that outside noise. If you choose ear buds, choose ones that fit in your ear well and are designed to block outside noise.

3. Take a sound break. Instead of always covering up sounds with even more sounds, try to block them out. You can use your ear protection, but even over-the-ear headphones block out quite a bit of noise when you're not playing music.

4. Find your quiet. This might be challenging if you live in a city. As hard as this is to say, you might just have to drive to find quiet, but it will be worth it.

Your quiet space doesn't have to be 100% free of the noises of modern life, but when you find your spot, the silence will drown out the noise and you'll know it…and feel it.

Where to next?

1. Something Fishy This Way Comes (p.102)
2. Get Dirty (p.395)

35

Stand Up For Yourself

by Roland

How sitting less will save your life, and how to start now without looking so weird

R emember the good old days when we thought 30 minutes of physical activity was enough for maintaining weight and good health?

Well, turns out that what we are doing the rest of the time may be way more important than what we do in those 3.5 hours a week when we go for our walk, hit the gym, or do a yoga workout.

See, our bodies evolved through moving constantly – movement was a requirement for physical survival, and between getting food, preparing it, securing shelter, socializing with our tribe, and running from danger, we used our bodies a lot. Kids have most of that innate movement instinct in them before they learn to sit still and "behave" in school. Yet, once education and jobs become our survival priorities, we leave our body behind, and it no longer participates in our daily grind for success.

Too bad nature can't ignore the effects of movement starvation. Your body very much notices and responds with weakening bones, widening waistline, slouching shoulders, and dwindling eyesight. Now do you think 30 minutes of walking a day can undo 8 hours of sitting?

Both to our detriment and advantage, the body adapts to what we do or don't do, not what we do with the best of intentions.

One meta-analysis of studies involving 800,000 participants shows that risk of heart disease and diabetes doubles for those who sit the most. You are 50% more likely to prematurely die if you sit a

---

lot. The good news is that you don't need to do a ton of activity to make up for it. Studies are showing promising results for "exercise snacking" – a fancy term for taking just short breaks from sitting.

An Australian study from 2008 shows that breaking your sitting for as little as one minute can have very positive effects on blood sugar regulations, markers of heart disease, and weight management. A recent study from New Zealand showed that moving for one minute at a higher intensity, six times per day, can have a more beneficial effect on blood sugar regulation than a 30-minute bout of exercise. Good news for those of us short on time, right? Improve fat burning, reduce risk of degenerative disease, and feel better, just by choosing to move more often.

Galina and I both spend most of our workday standing. In fact, 90% of this book was written standing, and we have been doing it for years. Many of our clients spend 50% of their day sitting and the rest standing, or they go back and forth. For our clients on a fat loss program, standing has sped up their weight loss, led to improved muscle tone, more energy (including no more mid-afternoon slump), and general improvement in well-being. You may have heard all of that before and thought that there was no way to do anything about it, with the limitations of your job. And that may very well be true – maybe your job does require you to be pinned to a chair and a screen all day long. But if you are allowed to go to the bathroom, there is hope!

Are you looking carefully into a microscope all day long? This was the case for one of our clients who lost over 100 pounds while working at her job. Every time she was done with a tissue sample, she would walk to the second floor of the clinic, then go back down to keep working. She would also drink some water. This is someone whose job was to tell the surgeon upstairs whether it was cancer or not. Her job was serious. Yet she made it a priority to take care of her health, so she found a way to take small breaks that didn't affect her work, and so can you. Your eyes, heart, bladder, knees, feet, and every single cell of your body will be grateful for it!

A sobering story comes from a client we first met in 2013. She had started a second job, but because it didn't cut into her exercise time, she thought it wouldn't be an issue. However, the extra time at the office cut her walking from 12,000 steps a day down to 3,000.

Six months into the new job she had gained 35 pounds of unwanted fat, all around her midsection. Wonder how that's possible? Walking does burn calories, but in addition, an important enzyme involved in fat metabolism – lipoprotein lipase – is produced only as a result of movement. The more sedentary you are, the less of this enzyme is produced, and the more likely you are to gain fat over time.

A study asked men to purposefully cut down on their walking. They went from 10,000 to 1,500 steps a day, and in just two short weeks they were metabolizing both fat and sugars poorly. Did they gain weight? You bet – all around the midsection.

It's easy to act on this information if you have a plan. Since all of you reading this have unique jobs and unique opportunities to do something about moving, here is a menu of options to choose from.

Stand

This can be as simple as standing each time the phone rings, to creating a standup workstation, to switching to standing meetings with health-minded colleagues. It can be as simple as standing for a minute, or standing for a few hours.

Fidget

But don't just stand. Once comfortable with your standing alignment, you can start to shift weight to one leg or the other, dance around, pace, stand on one foot, roll your shoulders, turn your head, and otherwise keep things moving. Fidgeters burn more calories than non-fidgeters, but also tend to be naturally lean, good sugar metabolizers, and generally more upbeat about life. Not a natural fidgeter? You can fake it till you make it.

> With the increasing popularity of standup workstations, models, celebrities, and executive hackers are being photographed standing at them, often in high heels. If you are planning to stand more, remember to keep a pair of flat shoes at your desk, and avoid the consequences that come from more standing in heels.

Walk

Remember the men from the study who reduced their walking and started gaining weight? It works in both directions. Walk more and walk more often. Walking a little every 30 minutes can be just as valuable as walking for 30 minutes straight. Go to a far copier at your office, make periodic trips upstairs if you work from home, or even do a lap around your house or block. I am sure you can figure out a way to walk for just one minute.

Exercise breaks

Depending on your workspace or sitting space, this can be as simple as doing 10 squats to your chair or a few pushups every half hour. We have some kettlebell-crazy clients who work at home and do kettlebell swings every 30 minutes or so. For the office yogi, a stretch that involves the whole body such as a downdog or sun salutation is also a great way to get some exercise in. We have created a whole chapter dedicated to office exercises, so if this is where you want to focus, please check out that chapter next.

Your tasks for this chapter:

1. **Stand up for yourself!** – This is an easy one! Your focus is to just stand when you can. It can be as simple as standing to take a phone call or trying a makeshift standup workstation, taking exercise breaks, or walking more. Fidget, if you like. For more tips on how to create a standup workstation, visit our website: eatmovelive52.com.

2. **Walk around** – Not necessarily far or long, but set a timer to walk for a few minutes every 30. Bonus points if you can swing a walking meeting or use a wireless headset to take a conference call while you're walking.

3. **Exercise breaks** – These can feel silly in a busy office, but there you can combine your walking breaks and exercise breaks. Can you walk to a distant conference room and do some pushups or squats? People who work at home have it easy. There's no one watching but your cat.

Where to next?

1. Explore Your Breathing (p.260)
2. Take Off Your Shoes (p.172)

36

Intermittent Fasting

*How learning not to eat gives you the ultimate
power over junk food and your craving for treats*

People fast for religious purposes, for meditation, for hunger
strikes, and to prepare for medical testing, but you might be
surprised to know that there are physiological reasons to fast as well.
Training your body to go without food for extended periods of time
can powerfully influence your metabolism, fuel your willpower, and
decrease preoccupations with food and eating.

When would you consider fasting?

If you are trying to lose weight

No matter what your eating style is, if your goal is to reduce your
body fat, then you need to figure out how to eat less. Taking in fewer
calories can be easier when you fast, and as a bonus, fasting improves
your insulin sensitivity, helping you use the energy you take in more
efficiently, versus storing it as body fat.

One of the challenges of reducing calories is that meals can be
small, and you might have to leave the table hungry. Think of it –
if you're going to eat 1,500 calories, it's probably more satisfying
to eat two 750-calorie meals than three 400-calorie meals and two
150-calorie snacks. Small meals also make it challenging to join
friends and family for social events, or even a normal-sized dinner.
Feelings of deprivation can lead to difficulty sticking to the plan.

While improved insulin sensitivity is a primary concern for those
with metabolic syndrome and type 2 diabetes, it also helps dieters.
When your food behaviors feel good and are also good for you, it's a
win-win.

278   EAT WELL, MOVE WELL, LIVE WELL

NO BREAKFAST, NO FOOD, NO PROBLEM!

Last summer we took a short hike in the hills above Pasadena, California, with our friend Lisa, her family, and their dog, Annie.

Galina and I don't always eat breakfast, so we started the hike on an empty stomach, knowing that lunch was coming up when the hike was over. Turns out we weren't listening very well when Lisa described the hike, and our short hike was over four hours long, and we hadn't packed so much as a snack.

Hours later our friends stopped for a food break and expressed real concern that we didn't have anything to eat. We explained that we'd spent some time learning to go short spurts without food (intermittent fasting), so we'd be fine. In fact, we'd each gone much longer without food than this, and we'd lived!

After the four-hour hike and a one-hour drive, we arrived at our late-lunch destination, and were able to make healthy choices and stick to our usual way of eating. Had we not learned how to do an intermittent fast before, we would have been miserable that day, and surely would have ended up overeating at the mere sight of food.

If you are curious about your relationship with hunger

Our relationship with hunger is complex. Many thousands of years of evolution have primed us to eat when food is available and be able to survive long periods of hunger. In the modern world, food is easily obtainable everywhere, with no real periods of hunger. Many of us eat just to eat, because of this evolutionary drive to avoid the next hunger period, out of habit, because it's dinnertime, or because of emotional triggers, not because we're actually hungry.

By creating shorter and longer opportunities to fast you can start to recognize true hunger signals as a need for nutrients, and train yourself to respond to that, rather than obeying every emotional or environmental trigger to eat. Many of our students report feeling empowered by fasting – able to eat when they are hungry and not eat when they realize they just want to eat.

If you want to help your body repair

Studies have shown that intermittent fasting might improve your ability to fight off some diseases, improve insulin sensitivity, and encourage your body to more effectively repair, reconstruct, and turn over its own cells. This process is called autophagy, which is a more palatable way to say "eating one's self," or at least one's own cells, to make room for new ones.

When autophagy occurs, it's survival of the fittest, even at the cellular level. The old, sick cells get eaten up, making room for new, healthy cells. Proper cell turnover is important to keep tissues healthy, and to fight off the incursion of diseased tissues that you simply don't want around. Studies show that this process can even improve brain health and memory.

Remember when life extension and calorie restriction were in the news? We saw the great lengths that people would go to for health and better aging. Fans of calorie restriction were seeking the autophagy that they believed was only available by eating just enough food to survive. The good news is that the benefits they sought are found in intermittent fasting, not just in eating less food. That means we can do better than merely survive. We can actually thrive.

How to fast

Learning how to intermittently fast is simple. On day one, you will start with a one-hour fast. That doesn't sound like much of a fast, now does it? Actually, all I want you to do on day one is to eat breakfast an hour late.

Let's assume that you have a fairly typical day. You sleep until 6:30

a.m., get up for a 7 a.m. breakfast, lunch at noon, then dinner at 6. In between meals, you might have a snack, but maybe not. Ice cream about 9 p.m., then it's off to bed about 10. My example is not likely to be your routine exactly, but it's close enough for you to imagine, right?

By my math, the time between ice cream and breakfast is ten hours. We need to extend our time-without-food little by little, bit by bit, until about two weeks later, BAM, suddenly we're fasting!

Ready?

Go!

Your tasks for this chapter:

Over the next two weeks, you're going to learn how to fast by making tiny changes each day and over time creating a shorter eating window. The shorter the eating window, the longer the fast, after all. I've built in three days of your usual style of eating, just in case you have an important event that comes up or you just need a break.

Here's an example – imagining you eat breakfast at 7 a.m. and your last snack is at 9 p.m. This is a 14-hour eating window and a 10-hour fast.

Day 1 – Eat breakfast one hour later at 8 a.m.

Day 2 – Eat breakfast at 8 a.m. Eat your last meal an hour earlier at 8 p.m.

Day 3 – Push breakfast another hour to 9 a.m. Eat your last meal at 8 p.m.

Day 4 – Push breakfast to 10 a.m. and keep dinner to 8 p.m.

Day 5 – Fasting break #1. If you like, eat as usual on this day, eating your three or four meals when hungry. You can continue on your fasting schedule, if desired, though.

Day 6 – Push breakfast back another hour – now at 11 a.m. If this is too close to lunchtime, you can just have a small snack to tide you over and have a usual size lunch.

Day 7 – Fasting break #2, if desired.

Day 8 – Breakfast is now at 11 a.m., but it's time to consider making breakfast a brunch. If you can get away with an early lunch, that's certainly an option. The trick now is to be sure that whichever meal you're eating is still normal sized. Eat dinner at 8 p.m. Now you are down to a 9-hour eating window – with possibly two meals and a small snack.

Day 9 – You're now officially skipping breakfast. Have lunch at noon. Have dinner at 8 p.m. and you are in an 8-hour eating window with a 16-hour fast.

Days 10 through 14 – Adjust your mealtimes so you are staying within an 8-hour eating window with a 16-hour fast. If you feel great you can push it to a 20-hour fast and even 24-hour fast on those days.

Day 15 – Take a break for one day and think about how many days a week you would like to fast going forward.

You've just spent a lot of time practicing the ability to fast without feeling like you're going to die. Don't lose it! For best results going forward, do one 16–20-hour fast once a week. I like to do mine on Mondays. It's a good way to kickstart my diet again, and get things mentally back on track for the new week.

There are some good reasons to fast longer, but 16–20 hours gives you a good idea of how a fast feels, and how it feels to really be hungry vs. just wanting to eat out of habit. From a 20-hour fast you can easily extend your fasting abilities all the way to 24 hours or longer if you want to.

Our friend Mark Sisson at Mark's Daily Apple has a great series on expanding your intermittent fasting. Mark covers weight loss, brain health, and more at marksdailyapple.com/fasting-weight-loss.

Full links to resources can also be found at eatmovelive52.com.

Where to next?

1. Don't Have a Cow, Man! (p.86)
2. Grocery Wars (p.15)

Level Up Your Vacation

37 *Take the vacation you deserve, survive it in style, and come home healthy, rested, and guilt free*

by Galina

When I was a young personal trainer and didn't have much grasp of human behavior, I used to dread my clients' vacations. Many of them chose to go on all-inclusive trips where they had access to unlimited food and alcohol. I couldn't tell them to stick to their diet and exercise habits, yet I felt like an even bigger jerk watching them throw away months of disciplined work and dedication.

Most would leave for vacation lean, light, and strong and come back heavier, sluggish, and disappointed. Yet, there was the rare exception – those families who planned vacations around sightseeing and exploring new destinations. Instead of spending 10 days at the pool bar, they spent 10 days exploring Prague, Vienna, and Paris. Instead of hovering around the dessert table at dinner, they would dance the night away and sneak in a chocolate croissant on the way home. They would go surfing and zip-lining, scuba-diving, learn how to fish or hula dance.

People who maintained their weight, positive outlook, and healthy habits vacationed differently than others. They had made a conscious choice to make the most of vacation time while keeping to some, though not all, of their health habits.

Before I introduce the common denominators of healthy vacation proficiency, let's look at the two most common types of healthy vacationer – you'll likely recognize someone you know. Maybe even yourself.

284   EAT WELL, MOVE WELL, LIVE WELL

The "screw it all"

This human can be seen ordering three appetizers and three desserts just because he's on vacation. Beer at 10 in the morning is totally legit, and the only way he will go to the gym is to make fun of his friends who "don't know how to relax." This split personality vacationer can be the most clean and pristine eater on the planet, but both paleo dieting and daily nature hikes go out the window when he lands at a resort.

Dear "screw it all" vacationer, while you work really, really hard to stay healthy when you are at home, your vacation style speaks volumes about how much it strains you to stay this disciplined. You like to loosen up, but your healthy body is not used to the amounts of food and alcohol you tend to enjoy on vacation; neither is it used to lying around all day.

Think about this: If you could be a little less strict with yourself when you are back home, allowing a day or so each week of eating foods you normally enjoy on vacation, it's possible that you won't be so driven to excess when you are resting.

Pay attention to how you feel when you are active and fit – notice the energy and joy surging through your body when you come home from a hike. Think of taking that same energy on vacation with you, explore new places, and immerse yourself in local nature and activities. Allow your body to de-stress. Indulge in some local foods, but stay mindful of signals of fullness and satiety. These new habits will merge the best of both worlds. You will be able to take your rested, strong, and energized self back into your daily routine and feel amazing for weeks ahead.

The "worry wart"

The flip-side of the "screw it all" vacationer is the "worry wart," who brings his own protein bars and homemade trail mix along for the ride. He can often be seen returning a salad because they forgot to put the dressing on the side, lecturing everyone at the table on the negatives of trans-fats in onion rings, and complaining about the lack of grassfed beef on the island.

Worried too much about the soybean oil in the salad dressing, stressed by the option of beer instead of heart healthy red wine, he finally snaps and ends up turning into a "screw it all," himself, eating everything in sight, yet not enjoying his vacation one bit.

Dear "worry wart," I know that the way you eat is a part of who you are and I love you for it, but when you go on vacation, the rules can change. Stores are different, and you won't have 100% control of your meals. Can you remember the time before you ate so strictly? What were some foods you enjoyed? Take a deep breath and remember that stress will take you out faster than conventional produce.

Traveling is a great time to work on being flexible, experimenting with dishes and exercise routines. Think of your friends who go to Paris and eat their way through the city, only to come back and discover they did not have any problems with the local food, but also lost several pounds. The next time you travel, find some opportunities to have things exactly the way you want them, and allow plenty of time and space for spontaneous dinners, unplanned desserts, and exercise sessions that just happen. Will you try sprints and push-ups on the beach with the kids instead of carving out hours of your day for training while everyone else is together playing and resting?

The 4 common denominators of healthy vacations

There is a third type of healthy vacationer, one who neither says "screw it all" nor worries about every little dietary detail. In fact, this vacationer treats the food and exercise on a vacation a lot like the food and exercise back home, only with more variety and a lot less structure. A vacation is not about letting yourself go, but about having fun, relaxing, and letting go of some stress.

This third vacationer follows the four common denominators of healthy vacations – forget perfection, be active, stay mindful, and choose wisely – even though he probably doesn't know he's following them.

1. Forget perfection

The minute you leave for vacation, perfection is over, but consider that perfection might be overrated to begin with. Vacation should be a time to relax, which is why you are taking a vacation in the first place, right?

Back at home, many people find themselves in food ruts, feeling stuck eating the same healthy foods, day in and day out. What better time to try new tastes than when you're in a foreign land with exotic food?

When it comes to exercise, some worry about losing their progress in the gym, but is that unfounded? Professional athletes are actually told to take time off lifting and training, just so they will come back stronger. Your vacation is a great time to try new exercises, sports, movements, and games. Being able to play is one reason why you want to be fit, isn't it?

You've been living this healthy lifestyle for a while now, so you might have to lower certain expectations and let some things go. If letting go is that tough, maybe the standards you set for yourself were too high to begin with, even back at home.

Sometimes perfection itself needs a vacation.

2. Be active

For most people vacation means being a bit more relaxed with food – whether it's cherishing the local gelato, or taking a cooking class with traditional ingredients. To balance out the excess calories and any excess guilt, be as active as possible, before or after your meals. Hike, swim, venture into a new exercise class, or visit the hotel gym for a quick 30-minute workout. Be especially focused on doing so before feast-type meals.

3. Stay mindful

Mindfulness, or paying attention to what is happening in the present moment – the thoughts, emotions, sensations, images, and behaviors – is a powerful tool. Whether you are resting in a hot tub, having your feet rubbed by a reflexologist, climbing a steep hill, or

---

WHY GO ON VACATION ANYWAY?

While a vacation can sometimes feel like it exhausts more than it refreshes, the data on vacations and our health tells us that they are definitely worth it!

Multiple studies have found that men who vacationed regularly lived longer and were less likely to die from coronary heart disease, women who vacationed more often were less likely to be depressed, and were happier in their marriages!

Vacations have been studied quite a bit, and overall, regular vacationing has been correlated with higher life satisfaction, better mood, lower levels of health complaints, less perceived exhaustion, healthier family dynamics, and the prevention of job burnout.

City vs. country vacations have been studied as well, and it has been found that people who take vacations steeped in nature had lower concentrations of stress hormones, lower markers of heart disease risk, and better stress levels than those who vacationed in the city. Feeling guilty about that vacation? Rest easy, and know that your vacation is paying off in better health and happier relationships down the road.

EAT WELL, MOVE WELL, LIVE WELL

simply spear fishing, keep all your senses open to the experience. It's hard to overdo anything when you can truly enjoy it!

4. Choose wisely

A vacation works best when it best suits your needs. Want to be closer to your kids and spend quality time with them? Then waiting in line in an amusement park may not be the best option. Instead, try going wild, and learn to build a shelter and start a fire. Which would give you more opportunities to talk, bond, and reconnect? Which would feel more relaxing?

What about the romantic times you miss with your partner? Will a vacation that's booked up with sightseeing buses and museum tours provide the time and space to really be together?

Here are some less common vacation possibilities that may provide opportunities both for adults who want to stay mindful of their health goals and kids who want to have fun.

Camping – You can make camping as simple as setting up a tent, or as luxurious as renting a space-age RV. The most popular campsites get booked months in advance, so make sure you pick your spot early and reserve it. National parks are a great place to start. The nation's top five are Yosemite in California, Glacier Park in Montana, Grand Canyon in Arizona, Great Smoky Mountains in Tennessee, and Yellowstone in Montana, Idaho, and Wyoming. If you live close enough to a coast, beach camping is great for camping newbies.

Beach house – Picture waking up to crashing waves and gorgeous sunrises. Imagine enjoying a martini at sunset, and relaxing in the sand while watching your kids bodysurfing. Beach houses give you a lot of flexibility to prepare healthy meals, while you are still close enough to other types of entertainment for kids and grownups alike. Many beach houses are big enough for several families, which allows kids to play together, so grownups don't feel like they need to be a constant source of entertainment. A mountain cabin can be just as fun if the beach isn't your thing.

Healthy cruises – You can choose from vegan, paleo, and low-carb cruises, yoga cruises, running and marathon cruises, as well as mind-body cruises in an industry that is quickly adapting to a demand for healthier options. And once you have signed up for a healthy cruise, you are all-in – from fantastic healthy meals to active pastimes and creating the kind of social contacts you rarely have the chance to on land.

Education vacations – "Flamenco, football and fun for all in Barcelona" or "Mount Rushmore, Crazy Horse and the Badlands"? Stateside or overseas? Organized family vacations are easy to find. The best part is you don't have to plan anything, just enjoy tons of fun and activities planned for you. Head over to roadscholar.org for a full list of amazing education vacations, and search by interest or location.

As we were writing this chapter we were coming to the bittersweet realization that a lot of our favorite vacation spots are far away or require a lot of special planning and considerable investment. For us, at least, doing an amazing vacation like this is only possible once every two years or so, so we have figured out ways to take shorter invigorating breaks that let us take a breather once every couple of months.

A weekend vacation – Have you considered leaving Friday night and coming back Sunday? How about spending that close to home? There are plenty of retreat centers, spas, lodges, hotels, and bed and breakfasts in close proximity to most urban areas, so you can also save yourself the drive. You can plan the activities ahead, and look forward to massages, hikes, yoga classes, or surfing while you are waiting for Friday to come.

Two-day city vacation – You can rediscover museums and local history by diving into a nearby city for the weekend. You can leave early Saturday morning and spend two days walking and exploring. The last time we did this we ended up looking for a hidden pirate tower and walked 30 miles over two days.

Hotel-room getaway – No dishes, no laundry, no cleaning up, no coffee to make in the morning. Room service. Candles. Chocolate on your pillow. When life gets crazy, going home to a hotel room for one night and waking up to someone else making you breakfast may be all you need to see the world with new eyes.

Three-day cruise – If you live close to a harbor, jumping on a ship for three days may be a great short getaway. What we love about cruises is that you have the ability to choose between many different activities and still stay on top of your nutrition. Great if you have kids, too.

Art day – You can dedicate a whole day to the arts. Start by looking up local museums and art classes. And various wine shops are now teaming up with art teachers to provide a next-level tasting experience: enjoy a glass of wine and create art in the company of like-minded people.

Farm day – Pick 20 pounds of strawberries, pet some goats, learn how to compost. Many local farms are open to guests on the week-ends, and a day spent exploring farm life, getting healthy organic produce, and socializing can be truly the best way to leave all your other worries behind.

Spa day – Start with warm ginger tea, jump in the steam room, get a facial, a total body massage, reflexology, soak in Epsom salts, and then have a light healthy lunch, and you can take on any task waiting for you on Monday. It's something you can enjoy as a single or with a friend or partner.

The staycation – Take a day off work and stay home. Instead of focusing on piled-up chores like cleaning up the leaves from the roof, bathe in the sunshine of your porch, pick up a book from your nightstand and actually finish it, order in delicious lunch, call a friend over and bake some cookies. Your home probably has every-thing you need to rest, yet you rarely have the chance to see it with vacation eyes.

Your tasks for this chapter:

Remember the four common denominators of healthy vacations – forget perfection, be active, stay mindful, choose wisely.

1. Picture your last vacation. Is there anything you could improve in terms of how well you ate and how active you were? Was it the best vacation for your needs and you family's? If you could do it over, would you do something differently?

2. Now picture your ideal next vacation. It's okay to imagine it as not perfect. In fact, it will help, but consider the benefits of vacationing and let go in the best ways possible.

3. Plan that vacation! If it can be your next trip, then go for it. Talk to the family, plan it, and book it! Use the lead-up time to get yourself used to the idea that nothing is perfect, nor should it be, whether it's on vacation or back at home.

4. Plan your next short getaway. Your dream vacation might be next year, so make time for some mini-vacations to tide you over. Mini-vacations are also a great time to practice letting go before that big trip!

Now, where would you like to go?

Where to next?

1. Food is Medicine (p.50)
2. Hanging (p.197)

38 Your Dynamic Office

by Roland

Yeah, we know sitting all day is bad, but what are you gonna do?

Sitting is to the body like sugar is to the teeth.

— Dr. James Chestnut

Is sitting the new smoking?

Sitting has been in the news a lot in the last year or so. Every one's talking about it, everyone's doing it, but other than talking about doing less of it, no one really knows what to do about it. After all, we live in a world seemingly designed for sitting. And boy do we make our chairs comfy!

We sit in chairs to eat, drive, read, write, watch television, listen to lectures, enjoy movies and theater, and even to exercise. Seriously, notice all the exercise cycles that let you get your cardio on while sitting and pedaling. Even a lot of weight lifting can be done while sitting!

With the exception of sleeping and our short walks to and from our chairs, it seems that most people in Western countries spend their waking hours on their butts, and it's being blamed for a variety of lifestyle diseases and conditions. Studies show us that cardiovascular disease, metabolic syndrome, obesity, and shorter lifespans in general are all associated with a lot of time spent sitting.

Why is sitting bad?

Sitting isn't bad, per se, but too much sitting, to the exclusion of so many other movements and positions *is* bad.

Our tissues require a variety of different movements and bone and joint configurations, and overusing some and underusing others makes some of our parts get too much activity, while others get none.

James Levine, a leading researcher at the Mayo Clinic, did a cool study with Jamaican office workers and farmers. Using "magic underwear" with sensors built in, he found that overweight subjects averaged 1,500 daily movements and 600 minutes sitting, while the more active farmers averaged 5,000 movements and only 300 minutes sitting. The less they sat, the more they moved!

To take the bad of sitting to the next level, consider that we've designed most of our chairs to put us into the same exact position: knees bent to 90 degrees, hips at 90 degrees, and our arms out front for reading, steering, typing, and eating. Then, with a nod to well-meaning ergonomics, we fine-tune our chairs to get our bodies into the position that hurts the least, so we can work harder and sit longer!

While it's true that special chairs and cushions, ergonomic keyboards, and strategically placed monitors can help you keep carpal tunnel syndrome and back aches at bay, the issues go far deeper than that. Too much time in this one, basic position, even ergonomically fine-tuned, keeps the skeleton rigid, in what amounts to a cast. Some muscles are casted in a shortened, chronically tight position, others are cast too long to be able to do their job. In addition, our cardiovascular system can also suffer when we are in one basic position for long periods. Sitting in the same configuration all day long creates overuse and stiffening in some parts of our arteries and veins, leading to premature aging, calcification, and varicose veins. The lymphatic system also relies on rhythmical whole-body movement to function, and if we are still, it gets sluggish.

When we do finally stand up, our backs ache, we're hunched over, and it takes quite a few steps before we are are standing tall and, hopefully, walking smoothly again. Often, before that recovery can fully happen, we're back to sitting once again.

The standing solution?

Can't we just stop sitting and do everything standing up?

New products to support standing at work are popping up everywhere, whether it's an inexpensive way to convert your desk to a standup version or an expensive, automatic desk that adjusts with the touch of a button.

These tools are great, but not always convenient to use or affordable, and in the workplace, come with stares and funny looks. Even *with* these devices for our desks, we still have to sit. A lot. Most meetings, lunches, and commutes still come with seats. There's simply no way around it, and with the "all or nothing" attitudes that most of us have, when we are faced with a choice we think to be futile, we simply give up. In this case, we just keep sitting.

Since the media latched on to it, so many articles have been published on the dangers of sitting that now we're starting to see legitimate warnings against *standing* all day! It's true, even if we did manage to replace most of our sitting with standing, our problems would be the same, only different.

What if it's not sitting, but sitting still that's the new smoking?

It's not merely sitting that's the problem, and just standing to work isn't the solution. There's evidence that it's the act of holding these positions too long and too often that's the problem. Sit still or stand still, neither is better than the other.

There have been many studies showing the importance of exercise and activity, but a study recently published in *Diabetes*, the journal of the American Diabetes Association, showed that short, periodic – but easy – walking breaks had the greatest positive effect on health markers. Other studies confirm this, showing that a cycle of sitting at work, broken up by very short, easy walks had dramatic and positive effects on blood sugar and insulin response.

The great news here is that this work/break cycle also contributes to productivity. The Pomodoro Technique is one popular method based on this finding; you work on one task for 25 minutes, then take a 5-minute break before returning to work. When you do return to work, your body and mind are refreshed and you are also ready to focus.

Merely swapping out sitting for standing is not the solution to too much sitting. We need to stop sitting *still*, especially for long periods of time. Luckily, this is a lot easier to do than an all-out switch from sitting to standing.

Ideally, you need to use a variety of sitting and standing positions throughout the day, change them frequently, and make sure to get plenty of frequent movement. It also helps to do a little light recovery work, like stretching and mobility drills, to combat all the chronic sitting that you've probably been doing all your life.

It's not difficult, but you do need a plan.

Your tasks for this chapter:

1. **Track your sitting** – Log your typical daily tasks in list form, and then go down the list, noting the position you're in for each activity. For example: Sleep – lying down; Walk the dog

– standing; Breakfast – sitting; Drive to work – sitting; Work – sitting. Keep going until you've logged your entire day. It should end with you going back to bed.

When you're done with the day, go back and circle or highlight all the sitting. Hold onto your log, because you'll want to look back in a few weeks to see how far you've come.

2. **Sit less, stand more –** Using the log that you just created, pick a few areas of extended sitting. Think about ways to do some of those tasks standing up. Take your laptop to a countertop, or read your email on your tablet, standing up.

3. **When you do sit, sit better –** When you must sit, try to find different seating positions, different types of chairs, stools, or even the floor. And check out some of the great tools we list on our resources page. A Swiss ball is handy for sitting differently, but consider adding something like a Backjoy to your chair.

4. **When you do sit, don't sit still –** Move 5 minutes after every 25 minutes of work. A Pomodoro timer app comes in handy for a reminder to move around. Remember, you just have to walk around for five minutes; get a cup of tea or something. No need to work up a sweat.

5. **When you're not sitting, recover from it –** A few exercises, a few times per day, will do wonders to help curtail the effects of all the sitting that you do. Take five minutes to do your calf stretch, double calf stretch, top of the foot stretch, t-spine stretch, door hang, and roll your feet. You can see video demonstrations of these exercises in the resource section at eatmovelive52.com.

Where to next?

1. Goodbye, Turkey Head (p.181)

2. The Best Things Come in NO Packages (p.129)

Furniture Minimalism

39

Or, "What do you mean you don't have a couch?"

I loved our couch.

Our couch was beautiful and comfortable, but Galina said she wanted a couch-free home. I love her and I trust her, so I believed her when she said the most important reason for couch-free living was health. I suggested that we could have the couch and just not sit on it. Later she admitted she thought the couch I loved was ugly, and that she was killing two birds with one stone. (I still say ugly couch was not ugly.)

Still, when we moved last year, I said goodbye to our couch.

The problem with sitting

Sitting is not bad; sitting *too much* is bad. Sitting the *same way* too much is bad. Even though a sofa is not the same as an office chair, the dinner table, a car seat, the toilet, or a bar stool, from a body geometry standpoint, they are very similar.

In this classic chair-sitting position, your torso is supported by your pelvis. Your hips and knees are bent. Your tailbone is usually tucked under, unless you are paying extra attention to sit with your pelvis neutral, and your spine has lost some of its natural curvature.

On a muscular level, the extensive time spent in these positions leads to shortening of your leg, torso, and neck muscles. You are also weakening your hip and core musculature. Higher up, the relationship, angles, and tensions between torso, head, and neck can mean compromised breathing and circulation. Stillness itself is damaging: your body needs your muscles to help move blood,

300   EAT WELL, MOVE WELL, LIVE WELL

lymph, and nutrients around – when you sit in the same position, those processes slow down dramatically.

Because you take this same position so often and for such long periods of time, you are also creating patterns of muscle overuse and underuse. Once you finally stand upright, those tensions and patterns don't just leave your body, but stay to influence how you walk, run, and play with your kids.

If you sit for eight hours a day at work, and then come home to sit more, aren't you adding more hours of the same patterns that contribute to your poor posture and physical tensions, aches, and pains? You bet!

There is a simple way out – whole-body movements and changes in sitting position can create stimulation for your cells, starved from hours of sitting at work. Those movements can be small (such as straightening your knees when you sit) or big (such as squatting down to the ground to get all the way to the floor).

How do you do that? To practice freeing your tissues from the prison of sitting every time you need to sit down, use something different from a couch or chair. Sit on the ground, on a short ottoman, on a pillow, on a ball – this will both change your sitting posture and introduce whole-body movement.

The more you sit on the ground, on floor cushions, yoga bolsters, and pillows, the more you will be able to appreciate the work it takes to do it. You'll notice the effort needed to get into and out of these new-to-you positions. You will feel the need to balance, calculate, plan movements differently. With these new positions, your muscles are doing a lot more work than they would just flopping into a cushy couch at the end of the day. Consider the work that goes into getting down to the floor and getting back up again. Hello, bone-building

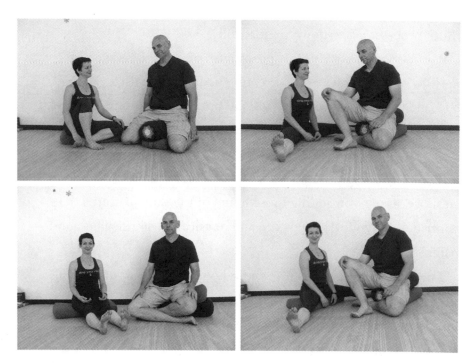

opportunities, muscle growth, metabolic conditioning, and nicer-looking abs!

Going from standing to seated on the floor uses new tissues and challenges your whole body differently, thus moving nutrients, blood, and lymph to and from areas that are commonly under-stimulated during the workday.

How easy is it for you to get down and get back up from the floor? Can you effortlessly drop down and come back up or do you need lots of help from walls and furniture? Studies have shown that the ability to get up from the ground without help, and how easy it is for you, is correlated with how long you might live. Even if "all-cause mortality" is not on your radar, the ability to be independent and move with freedom is key as we advance in age, athletic or not. You should be able to manage your own bodyweight against gravity

– basic strength is easily developed as you befriend the floor.

Imagine how frequently changing positions, from sitting to standing, from standing to walking, to sitting on the ground and getting back up again, sitting on a stool, then going for a walk, lying on the ground to stretch, and then a quick walk back home compares to most people's habit of sitting in chairs, car seats, and sofas all day.

It's not couch-free forever (unless you decide you love it)

Sure, we got rid of our couch, but we're not asking you to do the same. I'd love to hear that going couch-less for a while inspired you to eventually have a couch-less home, but that's up to you. What I want you to do for this chapter is simply not sit on your couch and chairs for a week or more and let us know how you feel.

There are other, indirect benefits to spending more time on the floor. I find that I use our foam rollers more, and that when I do watch TV, I stretch, and because I stretch more often, I stretch parts that I never used to stretch! Galina used to take a yoga class to sit on the floor and stretch, and now she just does all of that at home while we're relaxing together. You can literally enjoy moving your body together with family time and for us that is a win-win.

We recently hosted a dinner party, and our friends had a ton of fun stretching, foam rolling, and just lying around on the floor – since, well, there's no couch!

Your tasks for this chapter:

1. Sit less when you are at home and make a commitment to go couch-free for at least a week. I have to warn you that actually feeling the benefits of going couch-less can take longer than a week, so focus your *first* week on making your floor time more

comfortable. Pillows, rugs, yoga mats, yoga bolsters, cushions. I don't want you to be uncomfortable; I just want you out of your comfort zone.

2. After a week on the floor, you should be in the groove of going couch-less, so keep it up. Give couch-less living at least four weeks before deciding it's just not for you. After all, you've had a sofa your whole life, so give yourself time to reacquaint with the floor.

3. Invest in a floor cushion or some pillows that you like – it will look pretty, but also allow you to sit on the floor more.

For a tour of our couch-free home and video tips on sitting positons visit eatmovelive52.com. In the same section you will find out favorite floor-sitting cushions, too.

Where to next?

1. Stand Up For Yourself (p.273)
2. The E-Detox (p.382)

40

Are You Sleep-Deprived?

by Galina

*How to improve your sleep today, and an interview
with sleep researcher Dan Pardi*

*God has made sleep to be a sponge by which to rub out fatigue. A man's
roots are planted in night as in a soil.*

— Henry Beecher

I was a chronically sleep-deprived girl for most of my life. There
was no way to know that, with symptoms ranging from chronic
infections and fatigue, to lack of concentration, mood swings, heart
palpitations, and anxiety. I blamed diet, movement, stress, relationships, but never sleep.

When I moved to a foreign country and didn't work for a year, for
the first time since I was 18 I was able to get enough sleep and wake
up refreshed without an alarm. My symptoms disappeared.

Thinking back on the early sleep-deprived years, I falsely
attributed a lot of my symptoms to stress and my workload, an aspi-
ration for excellence, and an unhealthy affair with perfectionism.
Just one more client, just one more blog post, one more article, and
on the weekends, just one more party.

Stubborn body fat, sweet cravings, mood swings, and unstable
energy kept me company most days. If you asked me how I was,
I was doing "fine." When two major life losses hit me in my late
twenties, burnout hit me hard, powered by years of insufficient
sleep. Like most people, I had been well aware of the importance of
nutrition and movement in the prevention of disease, but sleep had
eluded me.

More and more studies are pointing to the powerful health-modulating effects of sleep. Researchers are looking at relationships between sleep deprivation and obesity, type 2 diabetes, chronic migraines, autoimmune disease, Alzheimer's, and different cancers.

Why are we sleeping less and why is the quality of our sleep suffering?

Modern life has made our days long and our nights short. We are spending an average of 20% less time in bed as compared to the 1960s. We are also "living" more of life under a light bulb and in front of the bright screens of TVs and computers, with some of our electronic devices coming with us to bed and completely changing our physiology by affecting our hormones.

"In searching for a link between stress and increased risk of cancer, it may not be surprising to find that women who have spent long periods working night shifts have an increased risk of breast cancer. However, the most plausible explanation here has nothing to do with stress. Instead, a shifted day/night schedule dramatically decreases the level of a light responsive hormone called melatonin, and depletion of this hormone greatly increases the risk of a number of types of cancer, including breast cancer."

— Robert Sapolsky, *Why Zebras Don't Get Ulcers*

Recently, a Harvard Medical School team released a study that compared reading paper books to reading on tablets and phones, how they each affected sleep rhythms. They found that reading via the electronically lit screens negatively impacted sleep quality, leading to fatigue the next morning. The screens' blue wavelengths of light were enough to suppress melatonin, and melatonin is a key hormone secreted as we approach bedtime. It does much more than merely help us snooze – it provides powerful protection from cancer and supports the immune system.

Sleep deprivation can also lead to increased insulin resistance, making us more likely to store fat and feel sluggish. It has also been shown to lead to overeating. One study revealed that when subjects were deprived of sleep for 8 days, they consumed over 500 calories more per day. They didn't change their activity levels one bit, either, and that's the recipe for weight gain.

Lack of sleep causes changes in hormones that regulate hunger and drive fat storage, but also changes our food behaviors. When tired, we tend to be more impulsive and choose foods that are easy, while providing us with quick, delicious energy. Tired, you are more likely to open a bag of chips than bake a potato, more likely to have a bar of chocolate than whip up a protein shake. So quick, so good, and so easy to overeat.

With lack of sleep, cortisol – a stress hormone – goes up, in turn lowering sex drive, messing up sex hormones, and wreaking havoc on the cardiovascular and metabolic systems. People who don't sleep enough are also more prone to infections. Those flus and colds that tend to come around Christmastime might seem to start with the holiday sugar overload, but the lack of rest and sleep might take the greatest toll on our ability to stay healthy. Lack of sleep is as much a holiday tradition as decorating the house and wrapping gifts these days.

What about cognitive abilities? Your memory and the ability to learn new tasks are also affected. Sleep is when our mind consolidates memories, and the less sleep time you get, the poorer your recall and retention will be.

If you could change only one aspect of your behavior, one that would elicit a powerful downstream effect on all biological systems and functions, it would be sleep. Why don't we see it? Why don't we get it? Could better sleep be the all-too-obvious, all-too-easy-to-miss, mundane measure we could take to improve our health and quality of life, but don't?

From our bright and sunny living room in California, Roland and I talked to Dan Pardi, a sleep researcher and creator of Dan's Plan – a program that helps you track and gain control of your sleep, eating, and movement habits, helping you create the health you deserve.

Dan, how much sleep is considered optimal?

Some important sleep determinants are duration and timing. Duration is how long you spend asleep across a 24-hour period. There are parts of the brain that are more and less active during different periods of your sleep. All states of sleep are important to the overall restoration process, so enough time spent sleeping is key.

Sleep can be all at one chunk, meaning you can sleep for 8 hours straight through the night, or get 6 hours at night and nap for 2 during the day. There are plenty of societies that do that and have good health and no cognitive performance issues.

Timing has to do with when sleep occurs. If you are used to sleeping 8 hours, and that sleep occurs from midnight to 8 a.m., but on the weekend you go to bed at 4 a.m. and wake up at noon – you're still sleeping 8 hours, but it won't have the same restorative quality as your usual sleep.

How do we determine when we've found our optimal amount of sleep?

When I work with people to try to figure out their sleep need, we first dial in their light rhythms and I ask them to give themselves an elongated period of time in bed – they may need only 8 hours or less, but I ask them to give themselves a full opportunity to get all the sleep they can and measure that. They do that for three weeks.

Some people say things like: "No matter what time I go to bed, I just can't sleep past 7 a.m." People can be misled about how much sleep you need because they wake up at their habitual time. The timing of your circadian alertness rhythm is strongly anchored. Even if you have additional sleep pressure, your wake drive will still alert you at your typical waking time. The best thing to do is go to bed earlier rather than plan to sleep later.

What are some effects of being sleep deprived?

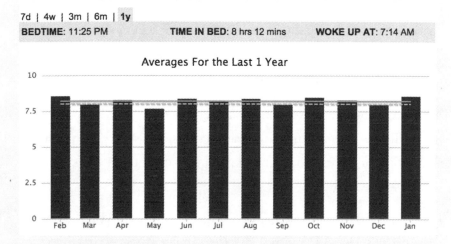

The big point for me is that it's a whole organism effect. Generally you can break impairment from sleep loss in two categories. Physiological, like alterations in blood pressure and changes in blood sugar. The other is behavioral, like loss of coordination and loss of motivation.

As you become sleep deprived, reaction time slows or you will miss things. Some of the most interesting research in this area is done by David Dinges, another sleep researcher. He is the inventor of the psychomotor vigilance test, which is a reaction time test that sleep researchers now utilize to test vigilance and alertness. You watch a screen for a signal, and as soon as it appears, you push a button as fast as you can. In the test, you are actively focusing on the screen, and you often still miss it. In a real-world condition this leads to accidents. We have a lot of lost lives due to car accidents – over 100,000 car accidents a year in the US. Not only that reaction time slows, but if you are trying to learn information, your ability to form memories significantly declines if you are not sleeping enough. Matt Walker, a memory researcher, found that not getting enough sleep on a regular basis led to remembering mostly the negative events. This can be an entry point into becoming depressed. We are seeing that people who don't sleep enough will more likely get depressed or develop OCD, etc. This is fascinating work that may help explain the connection.

The physiological consequences are significant, too. Metabolic impairment, cancers, and cardiovascular disease. Not getting enough sleep will cause the body to break, and that can be any physical system in the body.

Can you explain a bit more about light rhythms? What are some simple things people can do?

We want you first to focus on timing and duration. Spend enough time in bed to get complete sleep and make sure that your timing is consistent. Those are easy to track. The next step is to maintain smarter light rhythms. During the day the light outside is a lot stronger than it is inside. We have specialized cells within the retina that are sensitive to light and transform it into a nerve signal, and then it gets sent to the master clock. It tells the master clock what time of day it is based on the amount of light that gets into the eye.

We evolved with 24-hour light and dark cycles (circadian rhythm) and a lot of light exposure. Now we spend 90% of our time indoors, we are not getting much light outside and the light indoors is so much weaker. You may be surprised. Indoor, most light (measured in lux) is maybe 2,000 to 5,000. Outdoors it's over 100,000 lux. You will have a lot of photons entering the eye if you are outside. Inside, that message is so much weaker. A strong message will help anchor the circadian rhythm.

I was personally miserable for several years because my rhythm was not normal. I maintained a normal work schedule during the week, but I would go out late at night on weekends, and my 8 hours of sleep would be shifted, getting up late. I was in a perpetual state of jet lag.

A big problem today is that we acclimate to lack of sleep. You are not getting what is normal, yet you think you are doing fine. If you were to do an objective measurement of cognitive function, people would perform poorly, but their perception is that they are doing fine, they feel normal.

When it comes to getting outside light exposure, is there a best time or amount?

Luckily, there is a real Pareto principle happening here. Exposure to light will give you 80% of the effect in the first 20% of the exposure. One study looked at people who got 6 hours outside, and they saw that the first 30 minutes delivered 80% of the positive effect. I tell people to take all the opportunities they can to get outside. Aim for at least 30 minutes.

What about after dark?

After sundown, you want to mimic the natural environment by dimming lights in the evening. I make them dimmer and dimmer as the evening progresses. I also have a program called f.lux on my computer, which dims and blocks blue wavelengths of light automatically. About an hour before bed I will just go and read, and I read a paperwhite Kindle, which emits a very dim light and unlike backlit devices like phones or tablets, won't affect my rhythm. I don't watch TV an hour before bed and an hour before that I am wearing glasses that filter the blue light. I try to maintain that pattern and it seems doable for most people.

What about people who live at higher latitudes, where it's colder and the light is less strong?

Yes, people who live in those conditions don't get enough light – it's dimmer and also it's inhospitable to go outside. This sets up a situation for seasonal affective disorder. I tell people to get light boxes. A study in Antarctica showed that when they added extra-strong blue lights to this research station they found that people's reaction time and mood were improved with just stronger indoor light. You can buy something like the Philips goLITE and use that during the day.

Where does one start with all of this? Is there an order of importance to the interventions?

The big trend now is to do one little step to get one started. At the same time, a large change can be much better. I don't feel bad asking someone to spend 30 minutes outside, turn down the lights in the evening, and plan enough time in bed. Those three things are easy.

The problem with sleep is that it's mundane but meaningful – it's easy to overlook.

How does sleep environment play into this? Does it matter?

You want to sleep in a cool, comfortable room. Make it as cool as you can where it's still comfortable. It helps to facilitate the drop in core temperature. That's an important factor for the initiation and maintenance of sleep. Too hot a room will cause some insomnia or interrupted sleep. Blackout shades are great, but I sleep with an eye mask and earplugs and that reduces aspects of my environment that can intrude into my sleep. Light can penetrate through the eyelids, so if you slept in a lit room, that can interfere with your circadian rhythm. Neonatal children in the ICU don't develop as quickly, and we see that they have impaired performance in school at grades 3 and 5 and up until high school. This has lasting effects on our physiology.

Talking to Dan, I am grateful that we have implemented these changes, and grateful that we took the time to make them part of our lives. Your tasks for this chapter follow the order in which we started tuning in to all the aspects of natural sleep, per Dan's advice. This may take some of you a couple of weeks, others, longer. Take your time and enjoy becoming a better sleeper, even just one step at a time.

Your tasks for this chapter:

1. Start tracking. Find out how long you are sleeping. You can write in your journal, use a Fitbit or other wearable device, or use dansplan.com.

2. Like Dan Pardi recommends, spend 30 minutes outside (or with a blue light) every day, dim the lights or wear yellow glasses in the evening, and plan for enough time in bed.

3. Spend a few weeks trying to go to bed early enough to wake up before the alarm to see if you can find your optimal sleep. Remember that you might need to go to bed earlier, rather than plan on being able to sleep in.

4. Take things to the next level! Install f.lux or other blue-blocking software on your computer screens and other devices that you need to use after sunset. Consider taking an eInk or paperwhite Kindle or a traditional paper book to bed with you instead of bright screen devices. Consider earplugs, an eyemask, blackout curtains, cool air, and comfortable sheets for your bedroom, to enable deeper, sounder, and even better sleep.

Still curious about sleep? Consider doing some more reading. Great books to start with are *Why Zebras Don't Get Ulcers* by Robert Sapolsky and *Lights Out: Sleep, Sugar, and Survival* by T.S. Wiley. You can find a full list of resources and links at eatmovelive52.com.

Where to next?

1. I Have Needs (p.390)
2. Roll with It (p.230)

41

Sharpen Your Vision

Is relying on glasses when you're nearsighted actually shortsighted?

When the myopia has become stationary, change of air – a sea voyage if possible – should be prescribed.

— Henry Edward Juler, *A Handbook of Ophthalmic Science and Practice*

I used to wear glasses, but I don't anymore. I could not figure how I ended up growing out of my glasses in my early twenties, until I heard Todd Becker of Getting Stronger speak. Todd speaks about reversing myopia naturally by refocusing the eyes instead of using what is traditionally prescribed – glasses.

Then I came upon Jake Steiner, another myopia guy. The plot thickened. Jake makes a powerful parallel between eyesight and the food system. We have been using glasses to correct vision, without "seeing" the bigger picture, just like we have been using supplements to correct a lack of real food. When someone brings natural environment into the conversation, I listen.

How come when most of my English major peers got stronger and stronger prescriptions, my eyesight improved and I never needed glasses again? Here's why. Between my third and fourth year at university I felt burnt out and needed a break. I took a job as a water tour guide at Stingray City in the Cayman Islands. I took two semesters off and got to spend the winter in a bathing suit. But on the way there I forgot my glasses.

That year I didn't need to read much. No university, no library,

> "The way your eye works is that there's a circular muscle that controls the lens and which changes shape to give you clear vision at close and far distances. This is the 'ciliary' muscle. When you look at something far away the muscle is relaxed and it contracts to look at something close. The closer the point of focus the greater the contraction in this muscle will be."
>
> — Jake Steiner
>
> Just like we've talked about in other chapters of this book, any muscle that is tense won't be able to function well over time. Keep your pelvic floor too tense, and now it can't respond to the forces created by breathing, let alone jumping. Tense your ciliary muscles too long and you will get a similar result – a weakening.

no books. I worked on a boat and in the water, catching stingrays and showing them to tourists who flocked down from cruise ships. Coolest job ever. A sea voyage very much like the one Henry Edward Juler suggested in that quote. I used my eyes to track fish in the water, count passengers, and smile for the tourist cameras (check your old holiday photos – you may have a portrait with me!). All of those eye tasks were very different from reading. At night, I would walk, exercise, hang out at the beach, play pool, and dance. Again, no reading, other than the occasional fitness magazine. No Chaucer, no Mills, no Joyce...I was on a break.

Without knowing it, I had taken an eye vacation.

Eyes are not broken

Maybe you're thinking, this is crazy and there is no way I could have prevented my myopia by catching stingrays or taking long walks on the beach. Just like we didn't always know that the lack of vitamin C caused scurvy, there are still many areas of our health that we don't necessarily connect with environment or behavior. By enhancing your understanding of how eyes work, you may be able to prevent further weakening and damage, as well as take measures to protect the health of your growing kids or students.

Both anecdotal evidence and scientific studies now seem to suggest that it's possible to retrain your eyes back to full function. What if your eyes aren't meant to get worse and worse?

Epidemic of myopia

As early as the 1970s specialists were seeing the nature vs. nurture argument in the genesis of myopia. Dr. Francis Young, a researcher with a vibrant career and a huge legacy of studies, stated back then: "It appears quite clearly that myopia results from a continuous level of accommodation, and if one prevents this continuous level of accommodation from occurring, very little myopia, if any, should occur." In plain English, stop doing what you are doing and give your eyes a chance to do something else. This way little, if any, myopia will occur – behavior trumps genetics.

What is going on in the world that populations in parts of East Asia are reporting as high as 90% nearsightedness? If it's purely genetic, we wouldn't be seeing a rise of the condition in such geometric progression. In a study of indigenous Alaskans, Francis Young found that only 2 out of the 130 adults studied had myopia, while 60% of their children, who went to school, had developed the condition. The difference? Reading.

But I love my glasses

I look good in glasses too, but guess what? It's not worth the high tax of myopia. Luckily, I can still look sexy and fashionable in specs without it, even if all I get to wear these days are the blue-light blocking glasses that I wear before bed.

Myopia ranks as the fourth leading cause of blindness, and if you are nearsighted your risk for retinal detachment, macular degeneration, cataracts, and ultimately loss of vision goes up significantly.

Life today is nothing like the life humans were built for. We spend too much time using our close-up vision. First, when we are babies, we are given toys that dangle close over our heads. Then we go to daycare, which traditionally keeps kids within the limits of walls and fenced yards. Later it's off to school where our work is done with books, tablets, smartphone screens, and computers. At home, it's TV time. Most of our work, social interaction, and entertainment is all using our close-up focus.

The eye focuses much like a camera lens, and ours tend to focus best on far-away objects. Because of this specialization, when we do spend a lot of time up close, it comes at a price. Today, most of our time is spent looking at things close to the eyes – 20 to 25 inches is probably the average – for 8 to 10 hours a day. How many hours do you spend focusing on far-away objects versus close-up?

Outdoors – there is more to vitamin O than distance

So what do you find outdoors other than birds, trees, and mountains in the distance? Light, and plenty of it! That's right, one thing our indoor, confined working spaces lack is natural light.

A fantastic study from Australia looked at time spent outdoors and found that it was highly correlated with the risk of myopia. The researchers believe that a child should get about three hours of outdoor light exposure to prevent myopia, something that few kids get these days. In the study, a 40-minute after school outside break was enough to prevent myopia in a significant number of six-year-olds, cutting myopia rates by 25%!

We know the benefits of outdoor time go far beyond better

eyesight – socialization, vitamin D, probiotics, playing. While researchers are looking for even more great things that outdoor time can provide, you can take advantage of the veritable multivitamin that being outdoors – vitamin O – can bring now.

Why don't our eyes say something before they start breaking?

Humans, in all of our awesomeness, need mother nature to maintain our eye apparatus, just like we need varied terrain to maintain the health of our feet.

Nature didn't design us to spend countless hours reading and computering, so when our eye muscles become tense there is no discomfort or pain associated with it. Keep up your close-distance behaviors and the eye muscles will get weaker and weaker over time, with no obvious signals telling you to correct the behavior. You don't even know you have a problem until you stop seeing well, much like you don't always know your feet need help until you get an injury or a condition like plantar fasciitis.

CUT THE SUGAR FOR THE SAKE OF YOUR EYES

Sugar is the devil when it comes to eye health. Rapidly absorbed carbohdyrates are linked to retinopathy, macular degeneration, and cataracts. The warning is even greater for those with prediabetes and diabetes. See, the small blood vessels of the eye suffer just like the rest of our system from the damaging effects of blood sugar. In addition to minimizing the intake of sugar, it's also what we *don't* eat that can cause damage to the eyes. Make sure you have plenty of omega-3 fatty acids in your diet, from fish, krill, or seaweed. Load your plate with veggies and fruit for vitamin C and E. You best bets are citrus, bell peppers, leafy greens, broccoli, cauliflower, papaya, squash, nuts, and seeds. Become friends with lutein and zinc from shellfish, meat, and legumes, and vitamin B from organ meats, leafy greens, eggs, and dairy. Carotenoids, especially lutein and zeaxanthin, protect your eyes as well, so go for anything yellow, bright orange, and green.

Jake Steiner is of the opinion that most people diagnosed with myopia initially are experiencing a muscle spasm in the ciliary muscle, which is the muscle that focuses the eye. This allows the eye to remain stuck in close-up mode. Because the eyes are never corrected through proper refocusing, the muscle doesn't relax. Glasses then enter the picture, sharpening your vision by bringing the focal point to a different place on the eye, but do nothing to correct the muscle or the stuck focus. Think of glasses the same way you might think of orthotics. They are typically designed to compensate for a problem rather than to actually correct it.

It's not that our eyes aren't meant to focus close, it's just that we do it too much. Think of close-up viewing as sitting in a chair for your eyes. Is close vision the new smoking? Ha!

So do I just leave my life and head off on a sea voyage?

If you do, please take us with you – I could use a little vacation. But no, there's no need to head out to sea when there's so much you can do right here in civilization. Instead of forsaking all you love about the modern environment, see if you can make simple changes to some daily behaviors and give your eyes a chance to relax. Your vision could sharpen, and, who knows, maybe your eyeglass prescription will change for the better.

Replace eyesight-damaging habits with eyesight-improving habits

The two primary exercises that can improve your vision aren't hard, just hard to remember to do! In order to improve your vision, overall, it's important to exercise your vision close up and far away.

1. **Push your close-up vision** – When everything is in focus, your eyes aren't working out. "Print pushing" is a myopia

exercise that involves working out your eyes by reading outside of the normally comfortable distance. First, move your book, phone, or computer monitor back a bit farther than is comfortable for reading. Take it to blurry, then bring it back until you can just read it, but not comfortably. Spend fifteen minutes at a time reading like this, take a short break, and repeat. The process takes time, but it could be the key to stopping or reversing myopia.

2. **Look into the distance** – Make sure to exercise your long-distance viewing as well. Take frequent walking breaks and use the time to look at objects far away. Really look at them. Focus on them and their details. Riding in the passenger seat is another great time to exercise your long-distance viewing.

Jake Steiner also has a free course that covers these two exercises, and more, in detail. The information is in our resources section.

In addition to the above two exercises, it's important to alter your lifestyle so that you don't go right back to your old habits while you're still building your new ones.

Limit close-up vision after work – Stuck at the computer all day? Don't go home and get on your home computer or stare at a phone or tablet screen for the whole night. Instead, take frequent breaks from close-up vision to walk and look off into the distance.

Listen up – With podcasts, streaming services, and audiobooks, you can consume quite a bit of information without having to read a word. Listen up, and use your listening time to focus on distant scenery.

Don't look – By that I mean type without watching. I typed most of this chapter without looking at the screen. Instead, my eyes have been focusing at the mountain outside my window, the leaves on that tree, and at the clouds moving over the hills. If you can touch type, you should be able to type without looking. You might even find your typing speed increasing with practice!

Use fun and games to train your eyes – Play long-distance games like darts, horseshoes, bocce, lawn bowling, archery, and other forms of target practice.

Play eye games with your kids – "I spy with my little eye" is a great place to start, whether it's in the car or on a walk. Are there any other vision games you can think of?

I've successfully tried and implemented several eye-refocusing habits, and found them to be relatively easy. In fact, the hardest part was remembering to go outside on my breaks and look into the distance. A simple calendar alarm now reminds me to take my eye breaks.

Between the two exercises and the lifestyle habits, you'll be well on your way to seeing more clearly. Remember to head over to Jake Steiner's website and sign up for his free course, too!

Your tasks for this chapter:

1. Place reminders in your workplace to take a break from close-up vision. Take 30 seconds every 30 minutes and look off into the distance – a window or far wall is great.

2. Pay attention to your eye use after work. Replace close-up vision activities with going outside, or reading with listening.

3. Mix household chores with distance looking, such as looking outside the window when doing dishes.

4. Play some of the vision games suggested above with your kids or friends.

Where to next?

1. Let It Go (p.250)
2. Finding Your Health Tribe (p.374)

What the Tooth?

by Galina

42

What brushing your teeth can teach you about movement

I t's a beautiful morning. I walk into a dentist's office for a routine cleaning. The technician takes some X-rays and then comes and asks me when my last X-rays were taken. Three years ago, I reply. She tells me that the doctor will be right in.

The doctor informs me that routine cleaning won't cut it and I need to have deep scaling. There is local bone loss and severe local inflammation at four teeth.

In my mind I struggle: What are you talking about? I floss, use intradental brushes, I own a toothbrush that vibrates, beeps, sings, and flashes. I even own two different kinds of floss for those hard-to-reach places. I use essential oils to rinse.

I am told I need to double the flossing and brushing, refrain from foods that can enter the gum, such as nuts and seeds, and really need to think of seeing a periodontist to see if I need surgery.

I am thinking, "What the tooth?" I am only 35, and even given my genetics and poor dental care growing up in Eastern Europe, I shouldn't be dealing with this. I eat so well, move a ton, and chew thoroughly. Why do some people, who haven't been to the dentist in 10 years, enjoy perfect tooth health?

Fast forward and I am sitting in another office, 10,000 miles away, with a professor of periodontal studies, at the Medical University in Sofia. He finishes looking at my 3D scans, does some probing, examines all four "problem teeth" and concludes that I have some bone defects that need to be addressed through better hygiene and possibly antibiotic treatment.

"I can see you have fantastic hygiene," he says, "but that means nothing. We need to get your teeth clean in the right places, not just the places you always clean them.

"Brushing is a subconscious act. You learn how to brush and then you do it pretty much the same way over and over and over again. When you are told that you need better hygiene, you start to brush more.

"But let's define more – you can brush longer or you can brush harder. But that does not mean that your teeth will heal.

"No brush can get everywhere. There will always be places that get over-brushed and worn out and places that get under-brushed and form plaque and tartar. Usually those places are around teeth that become home to bacteria. Once bacteria settles, then pockets and bone loss occur. What I want you to do is analyze how you brush. I will recommend a regular brush, and a special soft tip brush that will allow you to enter the places that big brushes can't reach. Once every few days I want you to use a plaque revealing tablet in order to see the level to which you were able to clean the tooth. Usually, there will be a few spots that you don't brush habitually. You will take your brush and do whatever movements you need to do in order to clean those spots well. Then you will use the small brush, floss, and intradental brushes to clean the space between the teeth."

I am sitting there and can't believe my ears. My perfect tooth care story is practically the same story I get from my clients when they come to me with hip pain, low back pain, PMS and prolapses, migraines and chronic fatigue. They all tell me the same story: "I exercise. I eat well. I am a yoga teacher. I am a martial artist…but I hurt walking to the store."

The parallels were shocking. Just as my clients habitually moved in ways that caused their physical issues, my habitual movement patterns had now allowed my teeth to become ill.

I wanted to know more!

"What about mechanics?" I asked. "I can see in the 3D scans that my teeth are not entering the gum straight down. Is that some mechanical issue?"

Doctor Handsome looks at me and says, "We don't know what causes it. It could be mechanical. It could be autoimmune. It could be genetic. It could be bacterial."

Fine, I think. There must be somewhere I can start.

Over the next few days I brush and discover that these four teeth are ridiculously hard to clean – there are baby crevices in them that are hiding, and sticking the new itsy bitsy brush in there feels like spelunking. The picture starts to get clearer. I am battling a mechanical issue. On one hand my teeth are entering the jaw at an angle that is inappropriate. This is easy to fix with orthodontic treatment. But the other issue is an even bigger challenge – I have to teach myself how to brush again, checking to make sure I do it well, and then being persistent for months and months.

This was a few months ago. Since then, I've had dramatic improvement. During my last check-up the dentist told me she has never seen such improvement in gum health, not even with surgery. Here's to learning how to move my brush better!

Unless you are that rare individual who goes to the dentist once every 10 years only to find there is nothing to fix, you can probably benefit from better brushing mechanics.

Plaque coloring tablets are available at some stores, but they can be hard to find, so order them online and be done with it. After they arrive, brush your teeth exactly the way you always brush your teeth, then chew on a tablet. The dye will color any plaque left behind. Those colored spots need extra cleaning.

You can also use a small dental mirror to explore the hidden treasures of plaque, looking for more colored spots, and then address with your brush – do what you need to do to clear it.

Put a cherry on top by rinsing with a good mouthwash. There are several good brands on the market that you can find in the resources section, or you can make one at home for a fraction of the cost. Find the recipes at eatmovelive52.com.

Your tasks for this chapter:

1. Do the plaque-revealing experiment at least once this week. That will show you whether you need to brush differently. Keep brushing those long neglected spots, and then use the tablets to check them again.

2. Choose brushing movements that you have never done before. The tablets will help assure you've hit all the trouble spots, but just like hiking, new terrain brings new benefits.

3. Try a new mouthwash, or make your own using the recipe in our resources at eatmovelive52.com. Mouthwash is refreshing, but also great for rinsing away debris and bacteria that a brush can't always reach.

4. If you haven't been to the dentist in a while, make an appointment today. You will not only put your mind at ease, but also nip any possible cavities or gum problems in the bud. You've got options to try, should you need them.

Where to next?

1. Confessions of a Massage Addict (p.351)
2. Raw, Cooked, Juiced (p.134)

Read the Small Print

by Galina

43

Clean and detox your bathroom shelf, and yourself along with it

My hairdresser is going "sulfate free," my colleague has joined the "no poo" (no shampoo) movement, and now my dentist is posting online pictures of the homemade toothpaste she whipped up using baking soda, sea salt, and coconut oil. Is going all natural with cosmetics really that important, or should you investigate a bit more?

I've always been very selective with everything that goes on my plate – where did it grow, is it fertilized, with what, how long since it was picked, how was it cooked, is it nutritious enough? But somehow what went on my sun-kissed blond hair, foamed in my bathtub, and moisturized my skin was a bit off my radar. After all, you don't drink or eat your cosmetics, do you?

One of my doctors once wisely said: "Galina, if you don't believe me about cosmetics, go rub a clove of garlic on your feet. In just a few minutes you will be able to taste it in your mouth!" While I did go home and do it, and I could swear I could taste powerful garlic compounds in my mouth within minutes, I was not sure that it was a valid experiment. Scent itself is powerful enough to make you "taste" garlic, even when it's not present in the bloodstream. Being the healthy skeptic that I am, I had to look elsewhere for data that what you put on your skin can enter the body.

Enter my endocrinologist, a doctor with over 45 years of practice, who said: "Sure thing, dear girl, since we've had hormone creams, we've been able to help our patients so much better! Once through the skin, the chemicals can go straight to the blood and bypass the digestive system and the liver, so they are so much more potent and we can adjust dosages better!"

Okay, so if the pharmaceutical industry is all over a method that is more powerful than orally ingesting the same substance, I guess I can see why my dentist is concocting her own toothpaste.

Here is what I did when I first became aware of the potential toxicity of cosmetics. I realized that awareness was power and I chose not to be defeated. I chose not to freak out. After all, I had spent my whole life slathering on shampoos, pomades, petroleum lip gloss, lotions, and creams. So far, I seemed to be okay, but that doesn't mean I couldn't do better. Stressing about it was only going to make it worse, not better.

I went to the bathroom and embarked on a journey of reading the small print. About half an hour later, I was sitting next to a pile of shampoos, conditioners, bath salts, toothpaste, face serums, eye contouring crème, lipstick, and underarm deodorant, all destined to go to the trash. The only item that made it was a coconut-jojoba lip balm by some natural health company. Next stop, the natural food store to pick up some more natural replacements, but first I needed to learn what to look for in the small print!

Parabens – These chemicals are used to prolong shelf life, and studies link them to allergies, hormonal changes, and DNA damage to sperm and skin cells, where they react with UV rays. They even show up in samples of breast cancer tissues, leading some to believe that the accumulation of those compounds in your tissues may be a compounding factor in the development of fatal diseases. You can find them under the names methylparaben, butylparaben, and propylparaben, often at the very end of an ingredient list. Most of your shampoo, conditioner, makeup, sunscreen, shaving cream, face and body moisturizers contain one or more types of parabens.

Phthalates – Also known as Dibutyl phthalate, DBT, BzBP, DEP, and DMP, it is a solvent for dyes and a common ingredient in nail polish. It's been linked to developmental defects in babies, changes in fertility in adults, as well as liver and kidney damage. Multiple observational studies are looking at effects on diabetes and nervous system development. Check your nail polish for that toxin and get rid of it as soon as possible. There are many wonderful alternatives and also many organic nail bars popping up to meet the need!

BHA and BHT – Abbreviated for butylated hydroxyanisole and butylated hydroxytoluene, these chemicals appear in lipsticks and moisturizers. They are mainly blamed for hormone disruption, and have been found to damage liver, kidney, and blood in studies of mice.

Triclosan – It sounds familiar, because it's an antibiotic, but today it's also used in antiperspirants, deodorants, and hand-sanitizer. It's there because it's antibacterial and antifungal. You're most likely to find it in soap, sanitizer, and hand wipes, but it also appears in some toothpastes.

Perfume or fragrance – Perfumes are compounds that have a pleasant smell, or if odorless, have the ability to mask smells. They are used in deodorants, perfumes, creams, detergents, softeners, and are everywhere from your bathroom shelf to your laundry room and kitchen sink. They sound like a positive, but some can cause skin irritation, allergies, asthma, even neurotoxicity and endocrine disruptions.

Many companies have trade secrets around their ingredients so they don't have to list the type of fragrance that they use. Most labels will just say "aroma" or "fragrance."

Sodium laureth sulfate – or sodium lauryl ether sulfate – This chemical is what makes your bubble bath bubble and your shampoo lather. It's also what makes your toothpaste foamy. SLS has been linked to respiratory issues and it's one of the chemicals that accumulate in the marine environment.

There are many other chemicals that are known to cause irritation and disease, so I encourage you to do your own research online.

Just like with food, you can't be perfect. When you start to reduce your harmful exposure to these chemicals and products, you want to have some sort of a hierarchy – go for what you use the most or what covers the largest surface area of your body.

Some of the products we use the most would be shampoo and conditioner, body wash, body lotion, face cream, lip gloss and lip moisturizers, toothpaste, mouthwash, intimate hygiene products, bubble bath. Be cautious of anything you put on your child since they have delicate skin and weigh less than an adult.

You don't have to freak out over lipstick that you only wear once a year or a special Halloween nail polish since you use them so rarely. On the other hand, if you take sublingual and dermal applications of medications, you don't want to put possibly toxic and irritating chemicals in those places. Put these things higher on your list to replace.

Now that you have a clean bathroom shelf, what do you do? Do you join the no shampoo movement (called "no poo" by its fans)? Do you start washing your hair with vinegar? Just like with decisions regarding food, you can go a little way, a lot, or even too far in your desire to improve.

Before you rush out and spend a ton of money on all new, natural products, or run naked into the nearby woods, let's see if you already have some of what you need in your home. A few of the items in your kitchen are perfectly "edible" for your hair and skin, too.

Coconut oil – This popular oil can be bought for under $10 for a large jar. Use it to moisturize your skin and lips. You can add essential oils if you want to experience different fragrances or buy expeller-pressed coconut oil to go fragrance free.

You can also use coconut oil instead of mouthwash. After you brush your teeth, take a tablespoon of the oil and swish around your mouth for anywhere between 5 and 20 minutes. It might seem like a long time, but it's because coconut oil is so mild and gentle compared to most mouthwashes, which almost use brute force! Gentle or not, it can be an effective remedy if you have bleeding gums or sensitive teeth, and there are many anecdotes of its whitening effects, too.

Coconut oil can also be rubbed directly on your face as a cleanser. Just warm some in the palm of your hand, then massage on your face and use a warm wet washcloth to clean off the excess. This is what I do at night now and I love it.

Sea salt or Himalayan salt – You probably already have those in your kitchen, and you just have to move them to the bathroom. Fill a glass with warm water and add a teaspoon of salt to make mouthwash. This helps fight bacteria and leaves a pleasant fresh sensation in your mouth. It's also the perfect solution for those of you who use the Waterpick water floss. You can also use sea salt to prepare various natural body scrubs, mixing essential oils, coconut oil, salt, and sugar.

Baking soda – The small abrasive particles make a perfect ingredient for toothpaste. You can use it on its own, dipping your toothbrush in it. My dentist makes homemade toothpaste by mixing sea salt, baking soda, coconut oil, and clove essential oil. You can also add baking soda to your bath water for a relaxing and detoxifying effect on your skin. Want a deeper clean for your face? Mix baking soda and coconut oil as an exfoliant. The fine particles do the job perfectly!

Epsom salts – Those are probably sitting under the sink in your bathroom, just waiting to jump in your bathtub. Now that you've thrown away your bubble bath you need an alternative. A naturally occurring mix of magnesium and sulfate, Epsom salts can help you prepare a relaxing, soothing, and rejuvenating bath. They are a godsend for fatigued muscles and overworked brains. You can add scent to your bath by mixing essential oils in the water. My favorites are lavender and lemongrass, and sometimes I splurge and throw in several different oils at once.

Sugar – Coarse brown sugar makes some of the most popular body scrubs on the market. Why pay big money when you can make your own? Mix brown sugar with sesame oil, olive oil, or coconut oil, add used coffee grounds, a few drops of vanilla, and make yourself a delicious-smelling body scrub.

For all of your soap, antiperspirant, perfume, makeup, face cream, shampoo, and conditioner needs, head over to your local health food store and get a consultation with one of their assistants. It took me a few tries to find shampoo that I loved, but it's easy to take a few samples and experiment. And the body wash I use right now contains five different seed oils and apple pectin and leaves my skin feeling like velvet. Not one dangerous chemical in there, and it's the same cost as the mainstream product that I used before.

Are you ready for a new level of healthy? Not just inside, but out as well?

Your tasks for this chapter:

1. Use your journal to write down the products that you most often use, or those ones that cover the largest surface of your body. Use our list of the harmful compounds from this chapter to check the labels.

2. Try making at least one of the home remedies I mentioned above and see how you like it

3. Make a trip to the local health food store to replace toxic cosmetics with brands and products that are gentler to you and the environment alike.

4. Take your skin care one step further with one of our favorite authors – Liz Wolfe. Her help doesn't come in a bottle, though. With her Skintervention Guide she's created a complete education source to help you with your skin care from the inside out. Liz teaches you about the power of nutrition, and then suggests both foods and topical remedies that will help you sustain your natural beauty, from the inside out, and the outside in.

For a complete list of products I love and links to the companies that make them, check out eatmovelive52.com.

Where to next?

1. Eat Yourself Straight (p.72)
2. Take the Soda Challenge (p.38)

MIND AND BODY

44

Meditate on This

There are as many ways to meditate as there are people in the world

You should sit in meditation for twenty minutes every day — unless you're too busy. Then you should sit for an hour.

— Zen proverb

Vipassana meditation is a silent practice during which you practice self-observation, become aware of how life is formed in the body, and free your mind of suffering, pain, anxiety, and

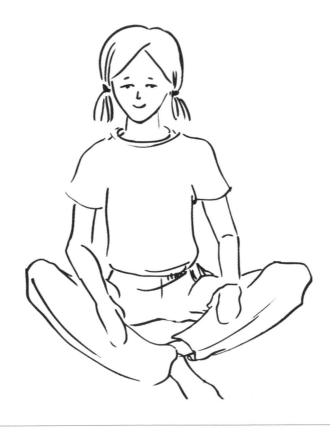

turmoil. The traditional course is ten days. Of silence. As in – you don't speak.

It might go without saying, but staying silent is hard. Geneen Roth, well known for her work in emotional eating and well versed in meditation practices, tells a story of a Vipassana retreat she went to in Joshua Tree, California. Just a couple of days into the silent retreat, Geneen was calling a private helicopter company to come and rescue her from the torture she'd signed up for.

Many people think exercise is hard, but do you ever wonder why activities like Crossfit, marathons, and bootcamps are so popular while quiet meditation (much less ten days of silence) is still something most people dread, and view as an activity for monks and hippies? Which activity is harder again?

Life today is a constant stream of stimulation – quite the opposite of silence or stillness. Texts, emails, notifications, sounds, lights, and activities pull us in numerous directions. We are constantly being entertained, involved, pulled toward something, or pushed away from something, asked to act now, click, purchase, return, evaluate, compete, and improve. Even the self-improvement business, with courses, books, and retreats, constantly pushes us to be better, perform, outdo. Usually right now, and with plenty of email reminders. Our already busy days are feeling shorter and shorter, and our mind's eye is focusing on the outside world rather than looking inward at our own needs for peace and, yes, silence. Add family responsibilities and dwindling personal time, and it's no wonder depression and anxiety, pain syndromes like fibromyalgia, and chronic fatigue are plaguing more and more of us. We simply never turn off. This "world overwhelm" is disrupting our physical, mental, and emotional health.

In nervous system regulation, what goes up, must come down. I'm sure you've felt it – you get excited, and then you calm down. You get upset, then you talk to a friend and come back to a state of relaxed readiness. If there are too many stimulating events and not enough time and opportunities to come back to relaxed readiness, stress, then tension, anxiety, and even pain may develop.

I am not suggesting you shut off the outside world and become a recluse or take a vow of silence like a monk. I am simply inviting you to explore this natural principle – notice the stimulation (what goes up), but also remember you have the ability to take a break from stimulation (and let it come down). Starting a meditation practice is easy. As easy as brushing your teeth.

First, think about how you'd like to experiment with meditation. I like to walk or sit, but you can also choose to lie, stand, or even dance, draw, or doodle.

Second, choose whether you'd like to focus on something specific or if you'd rather let your mind wander.

There are many styles of meditation with different traditions and schools. Some will have you do gentle exercise in nature, such as Qigong. Others will guide you to focus your eyes on a fixed point in space. A third might have you sit and let your thoughts or eyes go where they want to go, then observe how they shift to the next thought or object, like waves coming onto a shore, one after the other.

Third, set apart five minutes of your day. In those five minutes, you can start in the position you chose above – lie down comfortably, sit, stand. You can walk, dance, or doodle on a sheet of paper. Set a gentle-sounding timer, so that you have a distinct start and finish to your practice.

Choose to focus your attention on something, such as your breathing, while you draw, sit, or walk. Just observe it and don't change it. Notice how the air feels through your nose, how your chest and belly fill up, and notice the movement of the spine and muscles with every breath. Pay attention to subtle shifts in your body. Do you notice when something is feeling just a bit more relaxed, comfortable, better? When your five minutes are up, slowly return to your day.

If you choose NOT to focus your attention on anything, just lie, sit, walk, or dance with your thoughts, sensations, and feelings. As a thought or sensation or feeling comes, such as "my heel itches," just observe it and then notice how the next thought comes. Or "I feel fear." Notice as it comes, find the emotion in your body, then just acknowledge that specific emotion and sensation. Allow your attention to move to the next emotional, physical, or mental experience that it's attracted to. As you let that go, wait for what comes next and let that go off into the wind, like a cloud passing by. Your five minutes up yet? It will start to go faster than you expect.

Congratulations, you meditated

Like brushing your teeth, having a practice of meditation is not about the length or intensity of the practice. It's about frequency.

Do you have five minutes a day to check what's up on your social network, your email, the toothbrush, the newspaper? How about for meditating?

Multiple studies show the benefits of meditation. A 2014 systematic review and meta-analysis in the *Journal of the American Medical Association* looked at 47 trials with 3,515 participants and concluded that mindfulness meditation programs had a positive effect on anxiety, depression, pain, mental health, and related quality of life.

Many studies show an improvement in blood pressure, markers of metabolic syndrome, and stress reduction! Others are looking into meditation as a way to avoid medication and the serious complications that may arise from them. Could meditation become the dental floss for your mind?

Your tasks for this chapter:

1. Set aside five minutes of your day for your quiet practice. That's it. Choose the practice that best fits you.

2. If you feel like you want to jump further, you can find many guided meditation resources online. You can find links to them in the resources at eatmovelive52.com.

Where to next?

1. Move Like a Baby (p.207)
2. Let It Go (p.250)

45

Walk More Today

Baby steps to better health

Have you seen a baby walk for the first time? Ever notice how ecstatic the adults get – clapping and cheering? Then, as the weeks and months go by, the baby gets better, and just walks. No one notices anymore. No one claps. We take it for granted, because everyone walks, just like we always have. But do we still?

Historically speaking, ancient people walked a lot. While we can't know for sure how many steps they took on a daily basis, our estimates echo what we find in today's hunter/gatherer populations, where men tend to take over 14,000 steps per day. Westernized men, on the other hand, get about half that. Westernized women get even less, averaging only 5,200 steps per day!

We take walking for granted, even though we hardly walk at all, and it's taking its toll on our health in multiple ways. While ancient and modern hunter/gatherer societies can't be said to have perfect health, evidence shows us that the modern diseases of affluence, such as obesity, type 2 diabetes, heart disease, and other related conditions, were and are relatively unknown. A lot of their robust health is attributed to all that walking and higher physical activity levels.

Walking starvation is silent

Walking should be ranked right up there with eating and drinking, but unlike thirst or hunger, it may take months or years to first feel the side effects of not "consuming" enough walking. You may feel a lack of energy, different aches and pains, weight gain, and further down the road, increased blood pressure, varicose veins, joint degeneration, and bone loss. A not-so-silent side effect is being cranky, tired, and generally unpleasant to be around…but that can't be you, right?

Why don't we walk more? The most common complaint I hear from my clients is that they don't have time to walk, but they somehow do have time to drive to the gym, to the chiropractor, to a Pilates class, or to get a massage. All these things are valuable, they say, and suddenly there's no time left to walk.

What many people fail to recognize is that walking can actually replace a lot of what you do for your health already. It can save you from having a whole schedule organized around managing the aches and pains of a lifestyle that is walking-starved.

Walking. It does a body good.

Walking does you good in several ways: it moves and works your whole body, not just one muscle group or body part like when you hit up the weight machines at the gym. Since it loads your body vertically, with each step you take, powerful vibrations go through your skeleton, feet to skull, strengthening bones, muscles, and nerves, and stimulating organs along the way.

Think of it this way: you go to the gym and do three lower-body exercises, say three sets of fifteen squats, lunges, and step-ups. That is a total of 125 reps, right? Compare that to a one-mile walk, where you take 2,000 steps. This is almost twenty times the amount of movement you get in a lower-body workout session. Think about the volume of natural movement required by your muscles, ligaments, and bones to take 2,000 steps!

For bone building specifically, less does equal more when it comes to walking. The lower the impact and intensity, the longer and more often you'll be able to do it.

In addition to building bone, a 2014 study showed walking to be as effective as running for improving markers of blood pressure, cholesterol, and diabetes. Aren't these the reasons you "do cardio" anyway? If you only run because you think you need to run for health, then isn't this good news?

Roland and I run a weight loss program where walking is the number one recommended activity, and guess what? Our walkers are far less likely to overeat, they have lower stress levels, and enjoy more continued success losing weight than those who focus on more traditional exercise. I just measured a client who lost eighty pounds in one year, walking three to four miles per day, enjoying the great outdoors as she did her "cardio." Compare this to her best friend, who takes step aerobics and has hardly lost a single pound in six months.

Walk off the stress

If you're suffering from anxiety and depression, you will be glad to know that in studies, walking has been shown to be almost as effective as some medications. Be sure to work closely with your doctor before modifying your medication, but adding in a 30-minute walk out in the sunlight each day might just help you feel better. Wouldn't that be a pleasant surprise to you and your doctor?

Roland and I walk a ton. We each own pedometers that help us track distance and intensity. We got hooked on the Fitbit, an electronic, wireless pedometer, when I moved to the United States, and realized how much less I was moving here than back in Bulgaria.

In the US, particularly here in California, it's all about being in your car. People have phone conversations in their car, eat in their car, even watch movies in their car. Europe is all about walking – window shopping, knowing what new restaurant opened, greeting your neighbors, and getting drawn in by the fresh smells of the neighborhood café.

Once I moved here, I quickly went from walking six miles a day to two miles a day, and my waistline and mood started to show it. So Roland and I started wearing pedometers and looking for "walk-ortunities." I would wake up, go for a twenty-minute walk, later walk to get lunch, take another walk to the store to buy veggies, and often walk to see a friend who lives a few blocks away. If it was a busy day, Roland and I would walk and talk after work, discussing projects and how our days were.

While we often just walk, we regularly plan for our walks, too. We look at our tasks for the day and see where we can get them done walking, rather than driving. So where can you walk? Let's see.

Walk to the gym – Instead of parking right at the gym's entrance, park a five-minute walk away and warm up as you get there – listen to some motivating music, breathe in some fresh air. Ground walking is so much better for you than treadmill walking anyway.

Walk to the store – Need a carton of milk? You can actually walk to a lot of neighborhood stores. We have one within 10 minutes and another one within 30, so we can make it short or long. Need gum? Walk to a gas station.

Walk to a friend's house – Remember the old days when you would walk over to your friend's house and hang out for hours? If you are visiting someone within walking distance, leave the car behind. A glass of red wine with a friend can be quite healthy, but only when there's no driving involved afterward.

Walk to work (sort of) – If you need to be in the office, just park your car farther from work, walk to a local park for lunch, or head to a restaurant that's farther than your company's cafeteria. If you're the persuasive type, convince your coworkers to join you for walking meetings, too.

Make a walking map for your weekend – Weekends are the best times for longer walks. You can plan a hike, a picnic, or any adventure you like. If you prefer the city, map out a place to have breakfast, then walking distance to a movie theater, a skating rink, and a restaurant for dinner. Vacationers often find that they walk far more on vacation than at home; make your own city a place of interest and sightsee right there. Explore streets, paths, restaurants, shops, museums, galleries, parks, rivers, lakes, bridges, zoos, buildings, and other curiosities that you've wondered about. Kids love maps, too. Get them in on the fun!

The Walking Scavenger Hunt – Make it more fun for you or the kids by creating a checklist of items you want to see or find, such as: a very old tree, a hipster, a ladybug, a man on a motorcycle, five VW Bugs, a shaggy dog, a black cat. It can be a list of loud noises, such as a lawn mower, a Chihuahua barking, hip hop music, sea gulls, etc. Bring pen and paper and tick off what you saw, then when you get home, compare results with your friends or family. This walking adventure can also help keep your mind sharp, as you practice focusing on your surroundings instead of phones, tablets, and your daily grind.

Log your walking – A pedometer such as the Fitbit makes it easy to track your progress, but if you would rather keep a simple log, just jot down how long you walked in minutes, miles, or the measurement of your choice. Most of us need about 10,000 steps a day, on average, but you can do more or less on each day, as long as you average them out to hit your own weekly goal.

We all walk, but most of us don't walk nearly enough. Are you ready to take some steps to improve your heart, mood, bones, lungs, and energy levels?

Baby Steps. Adding even 10 minutes of walking a day is a great start. Just start. (You may not hear me, but I am clapping like a new mom does when she sees her baby stand up and walk for the first time!)

Your tasks for this chapter:

1. Use your journal to log how much walking you get on a daily basis. You can track time or distance, especially if you have an app on your phone or a pedometer. You can find detailed lists of the tools we like at eatmovelive52.com.

2. Once you find your starting daily and weekly averages, try to increase your daily steps by 500 to 1,000 or so steps, aiming for about10,000 per day, on average.

3. Over time, add more steps until you get to 70,000 or more per week. If you end up loving your walks, you may take up hiking, and easily hit weeks of 100,000 steps! Lots of steps are great, but there aren't many health benefits over our recommended 70–100k steps.

Where to next?

1. Your Dynamic Office (p.294)
2. This is the last time we pick for you! The Dynamic Office is one of the most powerful lessons in this book, whether you have an actual office or not. We all sit too much, don't we?

Confessions of a Massage Addict

46

by Galina

The healing power of touch is closer than you think

I t's Friday morning and I'm stuck in traffic. There are three meetings in my schedule before noon, a 15-minute break for lunch, then five clients in a row. I have my massage at 7 tonight, and I booked a long session, 90 minutes. This Friday is busier than usual, and I would normally get very tense looking at a schedule like this. Only, knowing that I am ending my day under the hands of my massage therapist makes today feel like a breeze. Four hours till massage. Three hours till massage. Two hours. I am on the table. The week is over.

Massage has survived and continues to evolve, because it's the most fundamental means of giving care, affection and aid between human beings. Its healing qualities differ from those of other modalities because massage confers its benefits through the character and healing intention of those who give and receive it.

— Noah Calvert

When I first started to get massages I was in my 20s and I viewed them simply as a way to get relief from the soreness and discomfort I suffered from long and grueling workouts. My low back and neck would feel so free and open on the days I had a treatment. Some weeks I would get two sessions, and some even three, and I had four different massage therapists that took care of me. One was great with neck, one with low back, one with hips and feet. I knew who helped me relax, who got me ready to be back in the gym, and who could really motivate me to watch the way I sat, stood, and walked. Over time, massage evolved to be a special time for me – a time when I didn't have chores, to-do lists, a time to be just with my body. I grew very curious about how different body parts felt on different days, and started to develop an awareness of the many detailed effects of massage. I found I had more space to breathe, think, digest, create.

How does something as "simple" as massage provide such great benefits as stress relief, pain reduction, and increased productivity and creativity? Why would every traditional branch of healing have a massage component? And are you missing out on something if you are not receiving regular massage sessions?

Enter the felt sense

The felt sense is the ability to "be in the world" not just through sight, hearing, smell, and taste, but also through feeling the world with your body.

I've learned about the many ways that a massage therapist can help you from Thomas Myers, fascia and bodywork educator, and author of *Anatomy Trains*.

1. Massage helps connect people to the "unconscious physical." Through skilled touch, the practitioner stimulates the brain to once again "see" or "perceive" parts of the physical body when that connection has been lost. This influences our ability to relax and contract the appropriate muscles, and to move with greater ease and freedom. This restored proprioception can often help you realize your neck was stiff before a massage, even though you had no clue you were tight there at all.

2. A good massage therapist can help you become more consciously aware of habits like holding your breath when receiving unpleasant news, or walking with one foot turned way out to the side. It's a cool feeling when you realize you can suddenly walk better, and actually feel what your yoga teacher means when she says, "Breathe with your belly." This lost brain-body relationship can be recovered through different modalities of movement, such as the Feldenkrais Method, the Alexander technique, Hanna Somatic Education™, and Restorative Exercise™. Enjoying a massage is an easy way to start, and is accessible without a special teacher or learning a whole new style of moving. There's always time for that later, just keep reading this book!

3. A great massage therapist can also serve you at a fully conscious level, such as drawing attention to how you stand, sit, or move, or by giving you valuable stretches to do at home.

There's also nothing like the feeling when you let someone take care of you. Lots of us have a hard time letting go and letting people in. A good massage can open that door, too.

As you think of massage, it may help to divide it into three major paradigms, again based on Myers's great work. One is relaxation – a time-out from life in a pleasant atmosphere, often with some soothing sounds or relaxing music. Touch improves your circulation, helps flush out metabolites, reinvigorates the senses.

The second paradigm is corrective – addressing specific postural or functional issues, returning your shoulder blade to its natural position or decompressing your achy hip. At the clinic where I work, the massage therapist works in conjunction with the chiropractors, to help the clients' adjustments hold long term.

The third paradigm, according to Myers, is one where the whole person is treated. Instead of asking what's going on in the hip, the therapist may also look at the ankle, knee, low back, opposite shoulder, assess the stress status, and take into account major life events happening at the time, or medical trauma from the past. In this view of the body, the goal is often to get the whole person to function at a higher level. While some of this may sound new-age, multiple modalities help the body integrate life experiences more fully and lead to a resolution of symptoms and conditions that are often not helped by traditional methods alone.

So, you may be wondering whether this massage thing is worth trying. If you've never done it, it's a good idea to ask your friends who regularly do massage for some referrals. Listen carefully about what they like with each practitioner and choose the one that suits you best. Just like with any type of specialist, it may take you a while to find the right one for your needs. That's a normal process of discovery. I've been very fortunate to find skilled and attentive therapists after only a couple of tries. And no massage is wasted. Each felt good in its own way.

There are many different modalities of bodywork and I will briefly cover a few, so when you are ready to venture into the magical bliss of Massageland you'll know what's right for you.

Swedish – This is the massage most of us know from movies and TV, where you see individuals or couples relax under broad and gentle strokes. This is a great massage to relax the mind and body, and to help you cope with the stagnant feeling you get from sitting too much.

Deep tissue – A deeper touch can affect layers of muscles and fascia that lie under the visible muscles. Chronic muscle pain and tightness can be very well served by these techniques and can give you improved range of motion in various joints and patterns of movement. Athletes often find deep tissue resolves their nagging aches and pains.

Myofascial Release – In MFR, the myofascial release system developed by physical therapist John Barnes, the therapist applies gentle and long-lasting pressure to areas of fascial restriction. The goal is to decrease pain and restore motion in areas that have been injured or damaged through misuse. A therapist may just hold or shake a limb to make its tissues relax and return to natural tone. MFR can be good in addressing chronic pain after traumatic experiences.

Rolfing structural integration – The goal of a Rolfer (unlike the goal of a movement educator) is to bring the body to a place where its relationship with gravity creates an optimal environment for the function of all organs and systems. Rolfing utilizes the manipulation of tissues in order to bring the head, ribcage, pelvis, and legs into vertical alignment. It's a very powerful modality and often resolves years of postural dysfunction. Although it takes multiple sessions to start, I have seen it work fast and well in clients of all ages.

Thai massage – This traditional modality from Thailand is over 2,000 years old. Sessions are performed on the floor, you stay fully clothed, and the therapist uses pressure and yoga-like movements to create a specific effect in the body. I find it extremely pleasant and revealing of my inner tension patterns. I relax fully into the hands of my Thai massage therapist, and come out feeling like I had a full-body workout.

Chi Nei Tsang – This method focuses on the abdominal organs and restoring a healthier state to the whole body. It combines gentle touch and breathing to deliver better health to the digestive, respiratory, reproductive, and lymphatic systems. If you've already read our chapter on digestion and elimination you know that Chi Nei Tsang is great for digestive complaints.

Maya abdominal (Arvigo) – Maya abdominal massage was developed by Dr. Rosita Arvigo. It is based on the ancient massage traditions of Mayan healers. The technique is very gentle. The therapist works on the abdomen and pelvis to promote a more natural organ position. It addresses back and pelvic pain, reproductive issues, and painful menstrual periods. The therapist also teaches you how to do your own self-care at home.

Shiatsu – This Japanese technique uses the pressure of the therapist's fingers. Like in acupuncture, meridians are affected in a way believed to improve the balance and health of the whole system. After a session you should feel relaxed and have a renewed sense of well-being.

Craniosacral – This very light-touch, hands-on bodywork helps to release tension in the structures that surround the brain and the spinal cord so that the nervous system can communicate more effectively. The craniosacral system, by the official definition, refers to "the membranes and fluid that surround, protect and nourish the brain and spinal cord." Craniosacral can bring relief for many painful conditions, from chronic back and neck pain.

Reflexology – Based on traditional Chinese medicine, this modality works with the zones on hands, feet, and ears that correspond to specific organs and systems. It promotes blood and lymph flow, and many find it helps with relaxation. One thing I love about reflexology is that it can work well even for people who are averse to being undressed on a table or being touched, as hands, feet, and ears are generally the main areas of contact.

Here I am, at the end of writing this chapter, wanting yet another massage, but which one will I choose?

Your tasks for this chapter:

1. If you are already getting regular massages, think about trying a different modality. You could ask your current therapist to try a different technique on you, or ask around for a skilled therapist in any of the modalities I suggested.

2. Do some research in your area to find out where the most appreciated and skilled therapists practice. You can do some reading online or ask friends for referrals. Start to create your own list of massage therapists that you love and trust.

3. Book your massage!

Where to next?

1. Are You Sleep-Deprived? (p.305)
2. Take the Eating-In Challenge (p.66)

47

Yoga is Not Just for Yogis

by Galina

Five awesome moves from my awesome dad so you can be awesome too

I
n recent decades, yoga has gone from a mystical practice employed by people who want to retreat from the world to a way to stay sane while remaining in the world.

For many people yoga starts with a class or a retreat, and then becomes a several-classes-per-week lifestyle. Others begin a serious and dedicated home practice. Some embrace the whole philosophy including the spiritual, moral, and dietary practices, while others stay strictly within the physical parameters, enjoying the various yoga poses and the fitter feelings that come with them.

My dad is of the latter group. Now in his early 60s, he's a martial arts practitioner, who in his late 50s became a personal trainer. He sees yoga as a way to practice a physical activity that brings him joy and gives him energy. Unlike many in the Western world, he learned about yoga from a small book, likely smuggled into Bulgaria during the Cold War. The book was passed around amongst people like my dad, who loved health and fitness, and craved learning about what was out there in the world. Many years later, the exercises from that tiny, secret book are still his favorite way to start each day.

My dad has been doing the routine known as the Five Tibetan Rites for as long as I can remember. He rarely misses a day and when he does, he says his energy declines and he knows he is missing an important part of his self-care.

I asked him to show us the five exercises and to tell us more about the book.

"It's really very simple. You have to start slow, doing each exercise only three times at first, and then carefully build your way up to 21 over time. These exercises influence your hormonal system, so you may find they rev your energy up too high. If that's the case, then you should play around with how many of them you want to do to keep your energy levels balanced throughout the day!"

Even without the mysterious story of how the book came to my father, the story of the Five Tibetan Rites is quite interesting. The tale almost sounds like folklore.

The small book my dad used to learn the method was written by Peter Kelder, published under the title *The Eye of Revelation* in the 1930s. Kelder told a story of meeting an old British colonel who had studied the specific movements while living with some lamas in India. The lamas seemed to have found "a fountain of youth," and through practicing the exercises the colonel had experienced many of the claimed health benefits, such as improving his youthful posture and growing his hair back without a trace of gray. In the 1980s, the book was republished under the name *Ancient Secret of the Fountain of Youth,* and now touted benefits that included looking younger, better sleep, increased energy, freedom from joint pain, weight loss, improved endurance, and a heightened sense of well-being and vigor. According to the author the exercises work through promoting flow of life energy through activating and stimulating the seven chakras of the body. The author explains that as we get older, that energy decreases, and as we practice the exercises it can increase again, bringing youthfulness back.

It is hard for me to say what the actual mechanism behind these exercises is and whether they work on some mystical level or not. Grounded in what I understand about movement and the human body, I can safely say that improved flow of blood, lymph, and electricity will positively influence the function of the major glands in the body. The endocrine system does have the power to affect all of our physiological processes – this will in turn influence our perception of well-being, resilience under stress, ability to recover from the demands of life, and, oh well, why not the growth of hair, like Colonel Bradford observed?

Curious to try the Five Rites? Below is a description that follows the book very closely, alongside some pictures of my dad performing them.

RITE 1

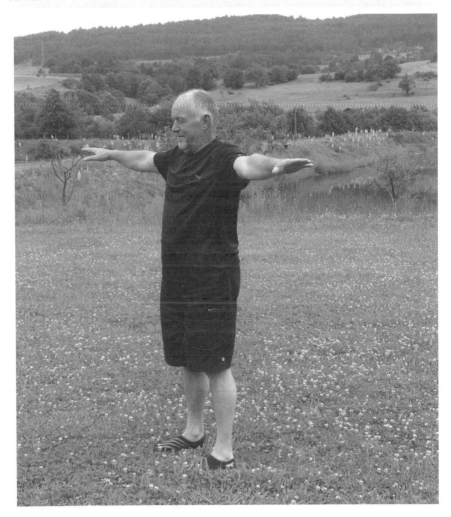

Stand erect with your arms outstretched and horizontal to the floor. Your arms should be in line with your shoulders, and your palms facing down. Spin, or turn slowly, always clockwise, inhaling and exhaling deeply as you turn. Start with 1 spin, stopping before you get dizzy, and increasing to 21 over time.

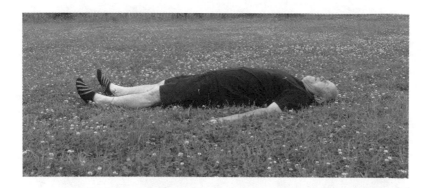

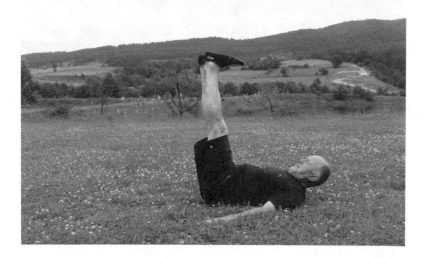

Lie face up, flat on the floor or yoga mat. Extend your arms down your sides, and place your palms against the floor, fingers together. Raise your head, bringing your chin to your chest. With legs straight, lift your legs as high as possible. Pause, then slowly lower your legs and your head to the starting position. Breathe in deeply on the way up, and exhale slowly and fully on the way down. Pause, relax, repeat.

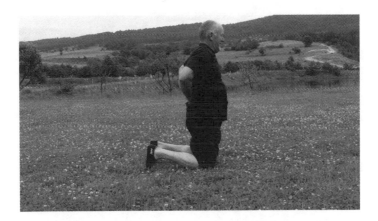

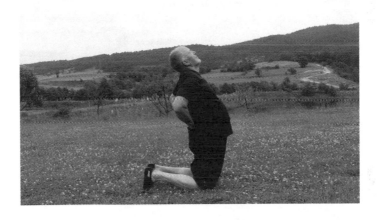

Kneel on the floor or yoga mat, with your toes curled behind you.
If this is too difficult, extend your toes so that the tops of your feet are
against the floor, instead. Body tall, place your hands on the backs of
your thighs. Tuck your chin to your chest, pause, then slowly extend
backward and upward, arching your back and making your neck long.
Use your hands on your thighs for support, and return to the starting
position, kneeling tall. Breathe in deeply as you extend, and exhale
slowly and fully as you return to the start. Pause, relax, repeat.

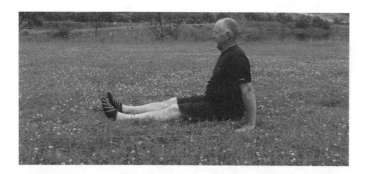

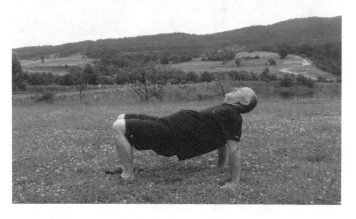

Sit on the floor or mat, legs straight in front of you, and feet about hip width. Sit up straight with your palms on the floor at your sides and let your chin drop to your chest. This is the starting position. Simultaneously extend your head up and back while raising your lower body off the ground, bending your knees and extending your hips until your torso is horizontal over your hands and feet. Think of yourself looking like a table top. Pause, tense every muscle of your body, and then return to the starting position by dropping your hips, sitting upright, and allowing your chin to return to your chest. Breathe in deeply as you rise into the top position, and exhale slowly and fully as you return to the start. Pause, relax, repeat.

EAT WELL, MOVE WELL, LIVE WELL

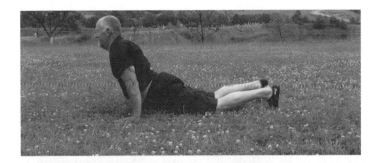

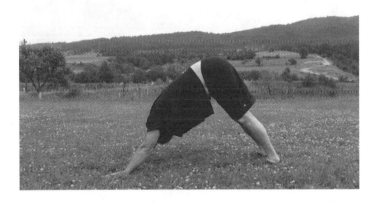

Lie down with your face to the floor or mat. Place your hands under your shoulders and straighten your arms while arching your back and tucking your toes under. Keeping the arms straight, bring the hips up toward the ceiling, and straighten the legs, forming a V. Most people will be up on their toes in this extended position. Lower yourself to the starting point, back gently arched, head and neck extended. If you're familiar with yoga poses, this one looks a lot like moving between the "up dog" and "down dog" positions. Breathe in deeply as you rise into the top position, and exhale slowly and fully as you return to the start. Pause, relax, repeat.

These classic, traditional yoga moves are designed to be simple but powerful. They are also flexible, even if you aren't as physically flexible as you'd like. Get into the positions as best you can, but never push yourself into a movement or posture you aren't comfortable in. Yoga is never about being perfect. Feel yourself get better over time and with practice.

What do you think? Do you want to try these exercises and see how you feel? They are performed one after the other, very much like the Vinyasa style of yoga. To me, they are a constant reminder that good mood and energy are just 10 minutes away.

Your tasks for this chapter:

1. Try three repetitions of these exercises over the next few days. Note how you are doing during and after them. Pay attention to energy, mood, creativity. Did your hair grow back yet? Wait a few months for this one!

2. After a few days, you'll be familiar with the movements, so try adding one or two repetitions. When you're ready, increase the number. One day, you'll get to 21!

3. Get yourself a copy of the book. New or used online, it goes for just a few dollars, and will provide you with inspiration and plenty of food for thought.

Where to next?

1. Good Fat, Bad Fat (p.77)
2. Now This Sucked (p.367)

48

Now This Sucked

by Galina

How to end a bad day well

I woke up late. Somehow I didn't hear my alarm. It was 7:30. My first client started at 8:00. That meant I had 30 minutes to get dressed, get my food, and walk to work. It takes 10 minutes to get dressed, 15 to get my food, and 25 to walk to work (I'd have to ride my bike). I texted my client and asked her to come 15 minutes later, then jumped into a pair of leggings and a dress. Screw the food at this point. I had a glass of water as I was shoving my crazy curls into a headband and jumping around the kitchen, one sock on, one off, toothbrush in my mouth.

Running down to the garage, I realized my bike was still at work, so I opted for my Razor scooter. Scoot, scoot, scoot, and by 8:00 I was frazzled and sweaty, but at work, and my day had only just begun.

Between clients, phone calls, and figuring out how to replace the lunch that I hadn't had time to make, by the end of the day, I felt like a lemon that had been zested, squeezed out, and thrown in the trash.

Was it a bad day? Yes and no. It wasn't bad in the kitchen-just-got-flooded, had-to-go-to-the-emergency-room kind of way; no one died, and people weren't stopping by with casseroles and looking at me with "those" eyes. This was somewhere between that and a bad hair day. The type of bad day that is pretty common for most of us.

Most of us know what to do with the really, really bad days. Car crash? Someone you love dies? We reach out for help, or if we fail to see it, people who care reach out to us. When my father-in-law recently passed, I cancelled my appointments, friends brought us meals, and relatives called, offered condolences, and visited.

It's the small sucky days that get you, because they are so common and often go unnoticed. They happen often enough to be "normal." But normal or not, it takes its toll. When you rush, skip meals, barely have time to pee between appointments, and have hardly taken a walk in months because you're trying to wrap up projects, the daily tax you pay on getting work and life done builds up. Somehow, just because it's a day like all others, and everyone seems to have days like that, you fail to recognize the toll a rushed life takes on your body. We've lost touch with ourselves.

I've had many discussions with my grandma and grandpa about the old rhythms of life. Once, their day started early – they would wake up with the sunrise, take care of the animals, the house, and then work in the field. The hard day would end at sunset, when everyone came in for rest, food, and sleep. Work was also seasonal – there were many months of the year when women would have time to be home, work on small and delicate crafts, dedicate themselves to family and children. Once the crop was gathered, men would spend more time planning the year, enjoying homemade liquor, and of course, making more babies.

Before the days of artificial light and the internet, sleep and rest took natural turns with going out and being active. People had rituals and customs synchronized with the light of the moon, the length of the day, the activities of the seasons, the availability of food, migration, and settling.

We've lost touch with this rhythm and its natural stress-relieving properties. Sucky days seem to repeat like in the movie *Groundhog Day*, over and over until one day you explode in rage or implode in depression, or just become numb to what once used to make you happy.

The first step in regaining control of your daily work and life rhythm is to recognize where elements of rest and restoration, gratitude and peace are missing.

The next step is to create a "sucky day menu" or ritual to follow when you've had a rough day. Rather than seething in anger and simmering in the poisonous juices of disappointment, you can gain control of how your body and mind respond to a difficult day. You can leave your battery drained or you can recharge it right away. What would you rather do?

When I finally got home that evening, the day was a blur. I put some scented oils in the diffuser and jumped in the shower. Out of the shower, I spent a leisurely couple of minutes drying off and choosing some soft and comfy clothes, enjoying the textures and colors, making sure nothing was too tight or compressive and that I actually liked what I was wearing. Then, I moved to the floor for a short meditation.

When Roland got home, we walked over to a nearby restaurant for dinner and just hung out and talked. On the way back I focused on feeling grounded and really enjoying the crisp night air, the smell of pine trees, and the freshly mowed grass.

Later that night over a hot cup of vanilla chai I sat down and wrote in my gratitude journal. I reminded myself of my client successes from the day, and I welcomed the prosperity of my business into my life. I took a look at tomorrow's schedule, turned off my electronics, and went to bed a little early so I could get in some needed extra sleep and start tomorrow with a fresh slate.

I was ready for my book and my bed, but I already felt as if each cell of my body had relaxed. I was ready to take on another day.

Your personal ritual

Developing a personal ritual for ending your day is a great life tool to master. On days when you feel like you have reached new heights, accomplished goals, and experienced the joy of victory, the close of the day can serve as a time to allow yourself to cherish the feelings, emotions, sensations, and significance of what's behind you. On days that leave you all wrung out and helpless, it's an opportunity to restore the flow of peace and safety, make sense of the experiences, and to build a stable platform from which to take on the next day.

I've developed various tools with my clients to support them in creating their own evening ritual. No matter what happens, I encourage them to be especially diligent and incorporate one or more of them if their day was challenging.

Grounding

You may have done grounding exercises in a yoga or tai chi class – it's a commonly taught practice that aims to guide your attention to your relationship with the ground, the seat, or the support behind your back. Get comfortable for your grounding exercise – I really like to sit in a chair or lie down for mine. Start by noticing your feet and how the ground is supporting them or your heels – allow the ground to come up and the legs to sink down. Picture roots spreading out from your feet through the carpet, down the building, through the soil, all the way to the center of earth. Try to tune in and see if any part of your body feels more grounded than another – see if you sense the right or left side to be heavier or more present. You can ground yourself anywhere you can focus, whether it's lying in bed, in your favorite chair, or on the living-room floor.

Meditation

Mindfulness-based practices are wonderful for those of us who feel stuck in a rat race. You can start with five minutes of quiet time a day. I was recently walking on the beach with one of my colleagues when she said she needed to hurry back to work. The sun was setting, so I said, "How about a minute of sun meditation?" We took a break to really take in the colors and warmth, the loving embrace of the sunset. The felt sense of peace and joy – it was wonderful. She mentioned how relaxed she felt, and how lovely it was to take that small break before heading back to class.

Gratitude Journal

Pouring your feelings onto paper gives you a chance to process the day. A gratitude journal takes that a step further, allowing you to pay attention specifically to the blessings in your life, and direct your thoughts to what is abundant, fair, and well, and away from what is hectic, crazy, and wrong. You can write as little as three words in your gratitude journal – kids, health, home? – but make it meaningful to you, and allow the feelings to really permeate you as you write.

Walking

Walking is a natural activity that is our birthright as an intelligent species roaming the earth for food and a better future. Nothing grounds and calms me more than a walk – in fact, I feel like walking has more benefit to me than all my other rituals at the end of the day. As you walk, you can also feel grounded, and use the time to clear the mind, like we do in meditation. The rhythmic action of walking, swinging arms and legs, has been proven to calm anxiety, lift people's mood, and increase creative ability.

Food creativity

Many of us cook only out of necessity, when we are hungry or need to provide our family with a meal. Coming home after a hard day and cooking is also a great way to relax. Preparing food can be a great reminder that the process can be more important than the end result – you can play with the ideas without having any expectations. I personally find cooking to be very relaxing, but use caution if you have a history of being a perfectionist in the kitchen, as this may not be your best way to end a sucky day.

Prayer

Whether you are an active believer or have your own way to be connected to a source of spiritual meaning and strength, find a means to give thanks and have faith in what is coming next. Our difficulties are powerful tools to chisel away at the parts that no longer serve us, and to strengthen our spiritual core. I'm also reminded that my difficulties are not always directed at me, but are things that all humans experience. This makes it easier to have a soft and compassionate heart, and to have mercy for others who might be less fortunate.

Dance

Dancing was always part of our ancestors' way to process stress and trauma – ritual dances, rain dances, ghost dances. It allows accumulated tension and reflexive responses to be released in a very fun and positive way! Whether you do a *Flash Dance* reenactment behind closed doors, or hit a dance studio or Zumba after work, you'll feel better when you are done.

Take a bath

The next time the events of the day are gnawing at you, take a bath! Set your phone aside, turn off the ringer, and ask your family not to bother you for half an hour. One or two cups of Epsom salts and a few drops of essential oils, such as lavender or clary sage, will relax your muscular and nervous systems, and improve mood and digestion. In order to reap the most benefits of a bath, make it a regular, even weekly, evening ritual, and observe the long-term effects on your mood, productivity, and creative drive.

Your tasks for this chapter:

1. Read through the end-of-day ritual suggestions and pick one or two to try right away. Aim to use one of these rituals at least four nights this week.

2. Keep a journal of what you like, what works, and what works with your lifestyle, then make a menu of these rituals to refer to whenever you have a hard day.

3. Establish a regular end-of-day, de-stress routine, but don't be afraid to mix it up. You have a whole menu of tools at your disposal now, and it's okay to change them up to keep it fresh!

Where to next?

1. I Have Needs (p.390)
2. Roll with It (p.230)

Finding Your Health Tribe

49

A good support system can be the key to success.
Luckily, finding yours doesn't have to be luck at all.

Karley is 35, works at a fashion magazine, and comes home late, tired and cranky from a long day. By the evening she's used up all her willpower on not punching her editor and not strangling snotty photographers.

She kicks off her shoes, changes into comfy leggings and a T-shirt, and heads into the kitchen to chop a salad. On the counter, a bowl of chocolates awaits. Her husband, a hipster chocolatier, brings home the extra pieces that didn't turn out perfect. Chipped truffles, gray-bloomed pralines, brittle bars. She glances over to the chocolates, then takes one, then one more, then 10 more.

This repeats every night.

Then there's Susan, whose boyfriend manages the Cheesecake Factory in town. Even though she's on a diet, he brings home pieces of cheesecake after work. She's a graphic designer and is on her computer late, catching up on projects, so she's still up, and struggling to stay awake while working. The cheesecake soon becomes her favorite treat before bed – it's just half a slice, after all.

Susan and Karley are a part of my women's coaching group – both struggle with extra weight. Today we're talking about their support systems.

"My support system?" smiles Susan. "It blows! My own family feeds me the very food they know I am trying to cut out! And my parents, well, all they talk about is babies."

"Mine doesn't blow. Mine sucks!" chuckles Karley.

As we burst into laughter, the sad undertones start to come up. And then there is some awkward silence that I dare to break.

"Change is a challenge. Everyone struggles sometimes. It's easier if we have a system in place, so when that struggle comes and we slip and fall, there is someone to catch us. Sorry to break it to you, girls, but even when they mean well, the people closest to you may not be the sturdiest branch on your support tree. If you have other branches, it will help. Let's get creative and see how to get you some support outside your home."

Susan and Karley are not alone. Many of us crave the support of loved ones when we are going through changes. And while your partner or parent or best friend may be there for you to console you after loss, or help you with job transitions and moving out of state, they may not be there when you are at war with a cheesecake, truffle, or pumpkin latte.

Susan, Karley, and I sat down with a cup of chamomile tea and a sheet of paper. I wrote "Building Your Health Tribe" at the top. We put ourselves in charge of creating the perfect support system for their health journey – a large tribe of like-minded individuals with a shared health value. For both girls the goal was simple: find people who will support them to eat well, move regularly, stay positive, and shed some unwanted weight in the process. In this powerful brainstorming exercise we came up with the members of an ideal health tribe. I present it to you below in no particular order, just like I brainstormed with Susan and Karley.

The healer – This is your doctor or functional medicine practitioner who not only has been to medical school and has a thriving practice, but also understands the power of nutrition in healing. They should be able to run lab work, do complex examinations, and make important choices when it comes to disease and dysfunction. You may be in great health, but it's nice to know you can reach to someone when your energy drops or your kid keeps getting ear infections. Want to find one? Head over to paleophysiciansnetwork.com for an easily searchable database of smart docs who are also nutrition savvy.

The touch therapist – Touching and grooming have always been a part of primate behavior – as humans started to organize into complex social systems, touching for health turned into organized schools of massage. We have deep longing for touch, from the first contact with our caregivers, to the caress of a loved one, to the comforting hand of a friend on our shoulder. Whether it's to move better, recover faster, or simply to relax, there's a massage modality for you; massagetherapy.com allows you to find a practitioner in your area.

The spiritual wo/man – Every tribe seems to have an old wise person who understands how nature, spirit, mind, and body work together. In an actual tribe they would have known your family for decades and remembered details that most have long forgotten. They can pray over you, sing songs of healing, and play music over your stressed-out body. In my life, that's my pastor and church counselor. I also have two friends who always stand by me when my spirit is weak. They have prayed with me through sickness, when I was stressed about getting my Green Card, and given me support when family members passed away. For you, it may be your meditation teacher, or that aunt who always makes you tea and has words of wise counsel. As you make a list of your health tribe, think of who's been a strong spiritual support for you, and who can be there again, or reach out to a local church or center for spiritual health.

The movement specialist – Once movement was intrinsic for survival. We would walk great distances to get water, find shelter, hunt, hide, gather, find a mate, run from natural disasters. Today, you could live your life with the click of a mouse, and get food delivered to your couch. But functioning optimally as a human being also requires movement – all your organs and systems depend on mechanical stimulation in order to thrive. Civilization has separated us from nature in many good ways, but it's also made it hard for us to see where our natural movement falls short. A movement specialist can be invaluable when you have chronic pain, want to recover from accidents, surgery, or injury, or just want to have an effective movement program to incorporate into your day. Develop a relationship with a local movement professional, such as a Feldenkrais teacher, physical therapist, chiropractor, or Nutritious Movement certified Restorative Exercise Specialist. They have their own network of movement specialists, and are usually happy to connect you with the one who's right for you.

The play team – How fun would it be to join a group of people once or twice per week to hike up a mountain, shoot hoops, or practice qui gong? How lovely to share a run, or the moments of deep peace, when the whole group breathes as one! I lead several groups, from walking to Restorative Exercise. We meet once or twice per week and we not only move together, but also we share life. We console the mom who sent a kid off to college, encourage a friend to keep moving after an accident, and give moral support when someone has emotional eating challenges. Local groups not your cup of tea? Join a virtual group, online. Forums and Facebook groups make it easy to find people with common interests and goals, not to mention dedicated social networks like Fitocracy. Still not finding what you want? Start your own group and "be the change you want to see in the world."

The shrink – My therapist officially told me we were done about five years into our weekly meetings, but made it clear that I can call her if something comes up. At the time, after many many many sessions, I was living the life I feel I was meant to live, authentic, happy, close to my purpose. I reach out to my therapist several times a year when I'm having a hard time processing everything that is happening in my life, which tends to come at light speed, it sometimes seems. My therapist specializes in Somatic Experience, which addresses developmental, physical, and emotional trauma through learning how to observe the body and its signals. Your needs may be quite different. You may not need a psychiatrist, psychologist, or Somatic Experience practitioner, but nearly everybody can benefit from a trained counselor of some kind – personal, family, marriage. Unfortunately, finding the perfect therapist for you can take time, but it's time well spent. You deserve to find the people who can support you. Whether it's to overcome addiction, understand emotions, or cope with difficult life seasons, therapy or counseling can help you live the life you want and deserve to live. It's often covered by your insurance carrier, so you can search in your network. For a list of Somatic Experience therapists, many of whom are also marriage and family therapists and psychiatrists, go to traumahealing.com.

The coach – Because you need someone to call "Coach." Wellness, nutrition, life coaches, business coaches, weight lifting coaches, happiness coaches, intimacy coaches – there is a wealth of choice out there for your needs. What makes a coach unique is that they have the ability to translate what your dietitian or doctor or psychiatrist says into actionable items. What sounds like gluten-free diet mumbo jumbo to you translates into a weekly food plan with the help of a nutrition coach. What looks like a huge obstacle in a relationship becomes an opportunity to get close to your partner in the hands of a relationship coach. You need a coach when you have a hard time applying what you know to what you do, but can't (or won't) do on your own. Roland and I are health, diet, and movement coaches, and coach individuals and groups, in person, remotely through phone and video calls, and in online groups. Do some online investigation and find your own coach to help you get on a path that is true to your desires.

The chef – Cooking at home has become a lost art, and while TV makes us think that cooking is reserved for polished, sexy chefs, the reality is that anyone can learn how to cook. Try learning from people you know who have mastered the art of cooking. Maybe that's your neighbor, your uncle, your friend from college, or a healthy chef at a local school. It really only matters that you love that person and what they have to teach you! Ask around or run a search on your local Yelp pages to find a teacher, or just ask friends over for a healthy cooking party! If you are in Southern California, call us – we teach cooking classes regularly!

The friend – Talking to Susan and Karley about change, we all agree that sometimes we just need a regular person to cheer us up and pick us up when we slip and fall. While a coach, a doctor, or a physical therapist may have the greatest skills and tools to help you achieve your goals, they aren't there at midnight when you are headed to the drive-through, or when you hear rumors of a lay-off at work. Think of a few people you know who are always there to encourage you in the right ways, pick you up when you're down, or are just naturally optimistic, open, happy, and healthy!

Building your health tribe is a fun brainstorming activity, but it doesn't really come to an end. Your own tribe will grow and change over time. You can keep jotting down the support you may need – a local grower at the farmer's market, a music teacher, a dance partner, a hiking buddy, a mountain biking team, a prayer group, a meditation group, a surfing teacher…

Your tasks for this chapter:

1. Make yourself a cup of tea, and open your journal or get out a sheet of paper. Go through the list above, and write down one or two of the tribe's members that you feel apply to you and that you have already or need in your life.

2. This week, do some research and find one new type of support – a walking group, a new doctor – and set up a meeting. If you feel like you need more, set up multiple meetings and sessions and see where that leads.

3. Find (or make) a group that can support you. Join one online or find a like-minded friend, then add more along the way. You might want to share your lists with your group, too. You've found your tribe, and they probably need you as much as you need them!

Where to next?

1. Are You Sleep-Deprived? (p.305)
2. Level Up Your Vacation (p.284)

The E-Detox

This is your brain on electronics

Do you need a break from technology?

When I don't have my cell phone on my person, sometimes it can feel like I am missing a limb because I feel so disconnected from all the people who I think are calling me, but really they aren't half the time.

— A Day Without Media,
International Center of Media and Public Agenda

I'm checking my email at the movies, and I feel like a fool. I have been looking forward to seeing this movie for months and here I am looking at my friend's cat video.

I feel like a cheat when I'm on a date with my husband and I respond to a text message from a client. Is the name of that Vietnamese restaurant that she forgot really that important?

And of course I feel publicly exposed when I am out to dinner with older friends who are not addicted to technology. They don't check their phones, both of their hands are visible on the table, and they seem to have better focus than I do, even though some are in their late 70s.

Since the internet has become a daily part of my life, being connected at all times and everywhere I go has become a given. Like fresh air, water, and food, wi-fi has become a nutrient that I demand.

In the early days of the internet, our connections would fail regularly, providing temporary chances to regain our sanity until they came back on. Now if our connection goes out for longer than a few

382   EAT WELL, MOVE WELL, LIVE WELL

minutes, we head straight to a coffee shop where a constant supply of warm and delicious wi-fi is always there to comfort us.

Today, even our phones are connected to email, Facebook, Instagram, and the entire internet. Weather, food reviews, calendars, maps, and apps are always there in our pockets, if not in our hands. At the touch of a button, I can reach out or be reached, immediately, constantly, and everywhere.

While today's technology is convenient, we might be paying a high tax for our always-on connectivity. Relationship problems, lack of attention to detail, and poor concentration are just some of the potential taxes. A habit of constant connectivity and electronic use have also been linked to worsening eyesight. To say nothing of the risks around driving while texting.

Most of us recognize that we're spending too much time with our precious devices, but because mobile phones, tablets, and computers are the modern standard for work and communication, stopping just isn't an option, even though many of us claim to be able to quit whenever we want.

The cost of empty pleasure

Like empty calories, there is such a thing as empty pleasure. Checking your email and social feed has an element of what's known as "reward unpredictability," a necessary step for the powerful release of dopamine, the same pleasure chemical that gets released when we're expecting a dose of a drug or activity we are addicted to. Once the chemicals and the behavior get linked, you just keep doing what any self-respecting lab rat would do and you keep pressing the buttons to get a dose of your favorite food or drug – in this case, a look at your social media feed or checking email.

But the satisfaction we get from such fleeting moments is not enough to feed our hungry hearts, which crave such things as physical touch, a look in the eyes, a smile returned, or meaningful conversation. As a result, we keep going back for some empty pleasure, never getting the fix we really need and missing important opportunities to really connect with the ones that could provide it. What a defeat!

Multitasking, or the cost of fragmented attention

Recently the marketing agency Tecmark published data that showed the average user picks up their phone 211 times a day. Some users tended to use their laptops and desktops for similar tasks, such as checking email, weather, calendar, or maps, an average of 140 additional times a day. Some of the participants admitted that they found themselves using their devices without thinking – checking social media or email.

The ability to focus on one task is something that is starting to elude us. After all, if the average person is interrupting what they are doing 350 times a day to check something, how much focusing time is left?

Even the ways in which we use our devices can take away from the tasks at hand and can cause attention fragmentation. If you were to record all the things you do on your computer in any one-hour period, it would probably seem insane: You watch a video for five minutes, head to a website to see who made the video, read their bio

> **THE IPHONE EFFECT**
>
> When behavior scientists observed people talking about meaningful subjects with and without a phone present at the table during conversation, they discovered that conversations without a phone present were rated as superior, more empathic and friendly, even among pairs of people who had closer relationships.

for three minutes, then head over to a link to their charity organization, read there for five minutes, then click the link to their Facebook profile page, find links to some recent news, watch two more videos. After all that, you finally get some writing done before getting distracted by an email.

…And that's just the first 20 minutes of the hour.

Finally, when you come up for air, you find that you received 10 text messages which have to be answered, and your to-do list hasn't even been opened.

Congratulations! You just carried out 40 tasks in 60 minutes. The bad news is that only 3 of them had to do with the actual work you initially set out to do. This has got to stop. Multitasking simply does not work, and multiple studies show it.

In a 2009 study from Stanford, we saw that people who considered themselves multitaskers performed poorly on tests that assessed their cognitive abilities. They were totally dominated by their colleagues who preferred to focus on a single task at a time.

Multitasking not only decreases performance, but it may lead to changes in the brain's cognitive control and its ability to filter out irrelevant information. All of this came as a bit of a surprise to the multitaskers, who considered themselves really good at multitasking, even when they weren't.

Your body bears the burden

Spending time fixated on a screen, whether it's TV, computer, tablet, or phone, means you are not doing something else – such as walking, enjoying play time, physical work, or being outdoors. As you know from other chapters in this book, sedentarism is severely punished in nature, and many of our systems can suffer as a result.

Time spent outdoors, preferably in nature, allows the eyes to focus

A DAY WITHOUT MEDIA

Can you go 24 hours without any media? This was the challenge presented to 200 college students by the International Center of Media and Public Agenda. The highlights of the study were hardly a surprise, yet were very sobering, as the students used many of the same terms to describe their media-free day that addicts of more traditional drugs use to describe their times without.

The students were more willing to give up television and newspapers than their devices, as they relied on them (and social media) for news as much as social interaction.

In addition, students equated going without their media to going without their family and friends in real life, even though they admitted that much of their personal communication with family and friends was typically via text message and Facebook.

far, get exposure to light, and to see what's happening in our peripheral line of vision. Time spent with a screen does exactly the opposite – the narrow focus strains eye muscles for short distance vision and doesn't let the eye muscles relax when it's time for long distance vision.

Myopia is just one easy-to-spot system failure, but negative changes are occurring at every level, from our craning necks to our failing hearts to obesity. Multiple studies have linked long screen times to increased risk of obesity and metabolic disease, regardless of the time spent doing physical activity later. It seems you can't just make up for too much time spent with your electronics.

The more screen time you log, the less likely you are to be healthy. This effect is especially pronounced in small children and adolescents, and excess weight and the epidemic of eyeglasses are just some of the red flags.

Technology can be a blessing, but it can also rob us of quality of life. Campaigns such as Screen Free Week, which urges you to go a whole week free of your devices, are popping up everywhere, making the public aware of the need to unplug and reset our brains and biology.

It starts at work, and never stops

For many of us, computers, electronics, and constant connectivity are part of the job. Clients need to reach you "right now," and your boss even more so. Nine to five, there is simply no rest. Years ago, when quitting time arrived, we left all that behind at the office. Today, we have mobile phones, home computers, and high-speed internet at home. Even if work stops, screen time never does.

Kansas State University researcher Young Ah Park encourages people to unplug from work activities after business hours in order to have more energy and productivity, but also higher levels of positive emotions and life satisfaction. Turns out, when you let your work take over all of your time, both home life and work life suffer. Yet, cutting the cord, or the wi-fi, isn't always an option or easy.

How dependent you are on technology will be influenced by your work and responsibilities, but even if you have to be plugged in at work, there are ways to minimize the damage. Here are some of the approaches we use with our clients, and ourselves, from easy to hard:

Give your eyes a break. When you are working at your computer or tablet, take a 1-minute break every 20 or 30 minutes, and look outside. It can be as easy as going to a window and focusing on a distant mountain, tree, or urban landmark. Looking at far-away objects keeps your eyes reactive and healthy, and helps prevent the progression of myopia.

Limit multitasking. Plan your day or project so that you work on the task at hand, while limiting your phone, email, and social networking time to planned breaks. Try the Pomodoro Technique in our Dynamic Office chapter and make yourself more productive and healthier at the same time.

Be sensitive to the use of technology after work, especially if you have to spend your workdays staring at screens. If possible, turn off email notifications after hours and on home devices and get in the habit of working during work hours rather than saving it for later.

Create technology-free zones in your home, such as the dining table, your bed, or even whole rooms, like the family room. This helps to limit screen time for the whole family.

Leave your phone at home or turn if off when you go to the store, on a hike, or during playtime with the kids. Practicing screen-free time in short chunks will eventually enable you to go without it longer. If you need to be reached for emergencies, try using your phone as a phone, and turn off your data when it's not absolutely necessary.

If you find that your fingers reach for applications like Facebook and Instagram without even consulting your brain, temporarily delete those apps from your phone or tablet. You can go back to them in a few weeks when you feel ready to do it on your own terms.

Try a whole day screen free. That's right, no TV, computer, game console, tablet, or mobile phone (other than for calls, if necessary). You might even make it an actual vacation day. A short vacation can be a great way to e-detox, and lets you concentrate on the things that you used to love before electronics showed up!

Once a year, try a screen-free week. You can learn more about it at screenfree.org.

Your tasks for this chapter:

1. Find out how much you use your screens. Get an average of your daily screen time. Much like logging your food, knowing exactly how much screen time you have is powerful. Then look to reduce it by 30 minutes a day and see if you can spend that time outdoors.

2. Try one or more of the suggestions above.

3. Discuss the screen-free idea at home and see what other family members think about it.

Where to next?

1. Squat Your Way to Health (p.239)
2. Drink Coffee. Not Too Much. Mostly Black. (p.95)

51 I Have Needs

by Galina

A peek at the health of intimacy, love, and desire

I recently got a card in the mail at my office. In the place of sender it said "secret admirer." Instant butterflies.

I was pretty sure the only secret admirer I had was my husband, so it was easy to guess, but as I opened it, the butterflies in my stomach were still fluttering their wings – then I saw his handwriting on the inside. On second look, I realized the envelope had our home address on it, which I had failed to see before I opened it.

There is something sweet and mysterious and forbidden about having a secret admirer. It leaves space for something to be discovered, waited for, explored, enjoyed. Something unknown and thrilling.

The card, sent by my husband, made me melt inside.

It's like when he goes on a business trip only to find my favorite writer is in that town, and gets a book personally signed for me. Or when I am traveling overseas and he sends me a sweater that still smells like him so I can cuddle with it on those cold winter European nights.

Those things warm your heart by touching you in a place only your partner knows about. It's what helps our relationship deepen and glow with a pleasant flame, daily.

Research for this chapter could have come from many places – counselors, therapists, books, and studies – but we thought it would be best coming from the heart and from our experiences as a family.

Our relationship was the long-distance kind. Not as in 3 hours away, but more like 22 hours on a plane. Between letters, emails, cards, books, perfumes, sweaters, spices, recipes, pictures, and yes, mix tapes, there was a constant stream of mail between California and Bulgaria, with each new day bringing an exciting opportunity to find that my boyfriend was thinking of me.

Thinking of me enough to go select a CD I would love. Enough to pour his heart out in an email. Enough to stay up late so I could wake up and say hello to him before work. Enough to stay home all day to cook with me on Skype – as I would make breakfast and lunch, he would make a snack and dinner. And then we'd eat together, like couples do when they live in the same house.

The ability to share thoughts, messages, yearning for closeness and real friendship over the distance of continents built a foundation for intimacy. When we got married and started living together, the rhythm of intimacy was already established – a coming together, a separating, and another coming together. Arriving, departing, saying hello, saying goodbye, a kiss after six months apart. Unbeknownst to us, we had found a rhythm that most couples lack, a rhythm that keeps us alive – apart and together, intimate, yet mysterious.

The definition of intimacy that most strongly speaks to us is "sharing that which is inmost with others." Researchers Helgeson, Shaver, and Dyer state that people perceive intimacy as feelings and expressions of closeness, appreciation, and affection. And of course it makes sense that closeness, appreciation, and affection are the pillars upon which to build a tower of love, warmth, connection, and even desire and lust. The more intimate and warm we are, the better. In our relationship we have found that there is a delicate balance between the intimate and the warm, and the separate and thrilling. Like the hot sand that needs the power and novelty of an unexpected wave to wash over it, lest it parch in the heat.

That wave is the flipside to closeness and vulnerability – it brings mystery, unpredictability, suspense, thrill, and novelty. It's the place for a secret admirer card, a surprise road trip, staying in a hotel for the weekend, or that trip to Italy and finding the gelato you had on your honeymoon. It's watching your partner talking to another woman at a party, and then looking at you and smiling across the room. It's drinking him in with your eyes as he sprints down the beach, chasing a kite. It's sending him off on a fishing trip with the guys – when you can be separate again, meet your selfish desires again, rekindle curiosity again. It's when you come apart so you can come together.

In *Mating in Captivity* Esther Perel writes: "Love and desire, they relate, but they also conflict. Love flourishes in an atmosphere of reciprocity, mutuality, and protection. Desire is more selfish — and we come with a whole list of injunctions against selfishness in love. Sometimes the very elements that nurture love block desire. The familiarity inherent in intimacy, the comfort we so desperately crave, can extinguish the flame of desire. My work with couples is to elicit strivings, longing, and novelty — to make interesting what is sufficiently available."

If you've ever moved to another country for someone, you know people ask why. What is it about that person that can make you leave home, career, relatives, roots, and make you replant elsewhere? I have had to answer the question "what is it about Roland?" so many times, I almost have an elevator speech about it.

"Every moment is interesting. Even the mundane is intriguing."

Interesting is that crossing point between being intimate and being separate. Between warm kiss hello and secret admirer card.

There is a chance you are reading this and you are not in a

relationship. We don't expect everyone to be in a non-platonic connection at the time of this book dropping from the sky onto your lap. We contend that the need for closeness, appreciation, and affection, as well as excitement and thrill, are engrained in all of us – whether single, in a thriving or just surviving relationship. You can deepen your connection with a platonic friend, a family member, start a new relationship, or use our inspiration to restart the fire of your current intimate relationship.

We invite you to explore your relationships through a few different activities:

Write a card – A just-because card, a miss-you card, a love-you-more-than-ever card. As you write your message, get quiet and think what makes you smile about the recipient, what makes your heart beat for that person, what makes you all warm and fuzzy inside. Now mail it to them, expecting nothing.

Send a memory – If it's cinnamon latte that you first bonded over, or a mission trip to Africa, send your friend or partner a reminder of a memory you have together. Mention when you think about it and how it makes you feel. It can be a spice, a scent, a picture, a piece of jewelry, a scarf, a special food, a piece of music.

Make a silly video – Five seconds may be all it takes to jump up and down saying, "I love you!"

Organize a surprise trip – Arrange a day, a weekend, a week, to steal your loved one or friend away. It may be super simple, like a day on the beach, or quite involved, like secretly finding a babysitter, or planning it out with your friend's whole family. I still remember taking my mom to the airport for a surprise birthday gift – she had no idea where were going to spend the week. That trip to Barcelona is still bright in our hearts, even though it was ages ago.

You can plan any gesture, gift, conversation, trip, according to your needs and specific situation. Think in two main ways: what shows comfort, sharing, affection, connection? And then what shows excitement, thrill, mystery, and unpredictability? As you plan how to reconnect and rekindle the relationship, think what's been missing. Is it the intimacy or is it the desire and thrill? And then bring it. Connect, separate, then connect again. Like the waves and the sand, one cannot live without the other.

Your tasks for this chapter:

1. Journal about a relationship that needs your attention. Determine if it needs warmth or thrill. Start to plan how you will connect to your friend or partner.

2. Take one action towards your desired outcome. Set things in motion, then keep things moving.

3. In following weeks, keep balancing the act of reaching with warmth and reaching with excitement. Notice how relationships flow differently and notice how your perception and experiences shift. Enjoy your old relationship, rekindled anew.

Where to next?

1. Ferment Your Food (p.124)
2. Learning to Cook from the Pros (p.31)

52 Get Dirty

I'm thinking pots, plants, shovels, and gravel. I don't know what you're thinking.

My first introduction to gardening was when I was six. Grandpa showed up with a bag of pearl onions. He pulled an onion out of the bag, placed it in the dirt, covered it thinly, and then had me continue to do the same. The game was on. Bam, bam, bam, they all went into the ground in what seemed like a matter of minutes. Grinning, I called Grandpa over to show off my work.

"They're upside down!" he said.

"What do you mean upside down?"

He showed me, and I did it over again, this time being careful to know which way was up and which way was down.

I've had to redo a lot of things in my life. Changed careers and schools. Moved countries. Married twice. Lost my business. Opened a new one. I often have to cook the same meal twice to get it right. I took driving lessons twice in a row, because I was not a natural driver.

Redos teach us about where up and down are in the world and that something you had a firm grasp on can be turned on its head in no time. In the garden, nature, like a patient parent, lets us deal with the consequences of messing up while allowing us to redo our work.

Have you ever gardened? What do *you* love about it? What are your plans for this gardening season? Can you walk outside and bathe in the glory of your garden – if so, I am happy for you and I am glad we share a love for the land.

Think you may be a black-thumb? For novices, I have a few ideas that will get you on a good green path.

Start small

What would you like to grow? A basil plant? A whole garden? A few roses?

Starting small allows you to learn without getting overwhelmed, and also grow a passion for more. If you grow 5 tomatoes, what would 25 be like, or 50?

If you are in an apartment, a few containers with herbs is a great place to start. Instead of starting from seeds, go to a local nursery and choose some young plants that you can tend to this season – preferably herbs you would eat. We have basil, thyme, mint, lemongrass, rosemary, sage, chives, parsley, and cilantro. You can start anywhere, though, and enjoy what you grow this season, planning to expand when you are ready.

If edible plants don't attract you, grab a gardening magazine and start planning your flower garden – depending on the climate you will be able to grow anything from forget-me-nots to cactus. Starting with a corner in your garden or patio can be affordable and achievable in a weekend.

HAVE YOU HEARD OF ECOTHERAPY?

The term was coined in the 90s and is also known as "green therapy" or "ecopsychology." Ecotherapists help people reconnect with nature and explore the relationships between humans and the natural environment, whether through gardening, being in the wild, bringing nature into hospitals, or working with animals.

Ecotherapy research is new and exciting, but *shinrin yoku*, or "forest bathing," has been around for a long time. Like other areas of ecotherapy, it uses nature to help people with depression, high blood pressure, PTSD, postoperative recovery, and more. You can see multiple ecotherapy resources at eatmovelive52.com.

Take a class

Roland and I took a class in natural pest control when we bought our aeroponic Tower Garden. Since we live in an apartment, containers and the tower are our only option to grow edible plants. We met other people from our area who were passionate about gardening, learned how to recognize the pesky leaf miner and how to kick an aphid's butt. We had a ton of fun and had a great growing and bug-butt-kicking season.

Most community centers have gardening classes. You can go online and find one pretty easily. This will also accelerate learning about gardening exactly where you are – what crops thrive, what the soil needs, and when is the best time to plant or harvest.

Grow what attracts you

Who's to say what you grow? At our home, arugula is king. I thrive on the bittersweet, crunchy leaves, mixed with tomatoes and goat cheese. In fact, I am off to make a salad right now and will be back to finish the section.

I have a friend who is obsessed with tomatoes to the point where he has more than 25 varieties and ends up having to give a lot of the crop away. The thrill of tasting a new variety makes it all worth it to him. As a beginner gardener, he just stuck the plants in the ground with no expectations and now it's his passion.

My parents love growing roses and they have more roses than I would ever care to get scratched by while picking or tending to them, but it makes my mom ecstatic to watch a new bud pop up and flower.

Chances are, if you love what you grow, you will love growing it.

I will leave you here, and invite you to think about the garden as a patient teacher in our restless world. Think of it as a place to rest from the urgencies of our day, experience it as a new way to respect food and the growing process. Think of your garden as a slice of Mother Nature's bounty that is yours by birthright and one you get to pass on. In the family, gardening is a natural way to pass on tradition, skill, craft, and recipes. If you garden, you can be endless. If you garden with others, that can be a powerful connection of friendship and sharing that extends all the way to the kitchen table. On an even deeper level, touching ground together bonds us as a tribe of humans that know how to survive.

Your tasks for this chapter:

1. Before you bite off more than you can chew, think about how much time you can spend each week, how much space you have, and how much sunlight you have to grow your future plants. All of these factor into your gardening choices. If you're a city dweller and want to grow more produce than your small or shady space will allow, consider looking into a community garden in your area.

2. For the experienced gardener: Step into your garden space. Look at it with the eye of a creator and see what you love about it – the colors, shapes, the way new buds are coming out. Feel the soil under your feet, hear the sound of the bees or birds. Get out your journal and spend some time dreaming about the next growing season. What would you like to have in your garden?

   For the novice: Play with the thought of starting a garden. Get a few herbs and plant them, talk to a few friends who may garden.

3. Start scouting for gardening classes in your area. Whether you want to grow herbs, fruit trees, flowers, or bonsai trees, there's a gardening class for you out there.

Where to next?

1. Intermittent Fasting (p.278)
2. Odds and Ends and the Anti-Cancer Soup (p.117)

In Closing

Congratulations! Here you are at the end of the book. Now what?

Eat Well, Move Well, Live Well covers a lot of ground when it comes to nutrition, exercise, and health. We wanted to keep each topic short and sweet, and we laid it out so that following along would be fun, no matter which type of reader you are. Which are you?

Did you choose your own adventure, following the options listed at the end of each chapter?

Did you read from start to finish, cover to cover, to see what was in store for you, and then plan out your strategy? Hopefully you're already acting on your favorite chapters, and building positive habits.

Or are you one of those people who can't take the not-knowing part? What's behind that door? What am I getting for my birthday? What's at the end of this book? How healthy will I be? What will they want me to do next? You probably read through the first few chapters, dove right in, and then flipped back here to break the suspense.

No matter your type, no matter how you got here, our message to you is pretty much the same: Don't stop. Keep up your momentum. Keep going!

No, you don't have to flip back to page one and start over. You've already learned so much, and come so far. This time you're going into this with your eyes wide open. You know which chapters had the most powerful effect on you and which might not have been needed, or maybe just not needed *yet*. You also know which ones were hard for you, or which ones were *too* hard right now.

Go check out the Table of Contents again. Take in the chapter names, and recall the topics. Remember how they helped you. How they made you feel better.

When we set out to write this book, we had no idea how hard it would be to limit ourselves to just 52 topics on better health. Truth be told, we wrote over 70 before we were told to knock it off. Even then we had to stop ourselves from writing more. Health is fun, especially once you really get going.

We went over the chapters and chose the 52 healthy topics that we are the most passionate about, that we thought could have a great impact on your lives, without turning your lives upside down. We learned a lot along the way. We even changed or perfected our own health habits as we wrote.

We don't expect everyone to adopt all of the habits in the 52 chapters of this book. You're healthier for each chapter you act on and for each habit you adopt. Some will have an immediate impact on you, while in other areas, you might feel like you're already doing great. Still other chapters will call to you later. You might not be ready to adopt that habit today, but perhaps one day you will be.

Your tasks:

1. Make a list of all the chapters. Use the Table of Contents as a guide, or just go to eatmovelive52.com and download the worksheet we made for you. Note which chapters had the greatest effect on you. Are the habits still with you today? Is it time to revisit one?

2. Note the chapters that you want to try again. Think about what stopped you last time, and consider whether you just weren't ready then or whether a small adjustment can make the

new habit fit better with your life. Never let perfection stand in the way of progress.

3. Circle the chapters you loved, cross out the ones you don't need, and make plenty of notes on what you want to do next as you choose your own health path.

4. Journal. If you started a paper or electronic journal when you first cracked opened this book, you have a record of your experience. Go back to your list of chapters and notice how you answered those basic questions back then. What spoke to you, and how can this help you now or later?

Where to next?

On our website we have outlined many other steps for most chapters, from recipes and tips, to articles and books, video resources for the exercises, interviews with experts, and ways to find professionals in your area.

As you head out to explore, you will find that each chapter in our book is an invitation and introduction to a whole new world, ready to be explored. Venture out, and have fun!

Stop by eatmovelive52.com and connect with us and others like you. Stay in touch, and let's Eat Well, Move Well, and Live Well together!

Roland & Galina

REFERENCES

3. Slow Down Your Meals

Alicja, M.B. et al. "Consumption of a Diet Low in Advanced Glycation End Products for 4 Weeks Improves Insulin Sensitivity in Overweight Women." *Diabetes Care* 2014;37(1):88-95. doi: 10.2337/dc13-0842.

Dalena, J. et al. "Pilot study: Mindful Eating and Living (MEAL): Weight, eating behavior, and psychological outcomes associated with a mindfulness-based intervention for people with obesity." *Complementary Therapies in Medicine* 2010 Dec;18(6):260-4. doi: 10.1016/j.ctim.2010.09.008

"The Harris Poll® #82," November 13, 2013, http://www.theharrispoll.com/health-and-life/Are_Americans_Still_Serving_Up_Family_Dinners_.htmlx

Tanihara, S. et al. "Retrospective longitudinal study on the relationship between 8-year weight change and current eating speed." *Appetite* 2011 Aug;57(1):179-83. doi: 10.1016/j.appet.2011.04.017

Radzevi ien , L. and Ostrauskas, R. "Fast eating and the risk of type

2 diabetes mellitus: A case-control study." *Clinical Nutrition* 2013 Apr;32(2):232-5. doi: 10.1016/j.clnu.2012.06.013

5. Take the Soda Challenge

"Fact sheet: Sugary drink supersizing and the obesity epidemic, Department of Nutrition at Harvard School of Public Health," http://www.hsph.harvard.edu/nutritionsource/sugary-drinks-fact-sheet/

Pan, A. and Hu, F.B. "Effects of carbohydrates on satiety: differences between liquid and solid food." *Current Opinion in Clinical Nutrition & Metabolic Care.* 2011 Jul;14(4):385-90. doi:10.1097/MCO.0b013e328346df36.

6. Detox Your Pantry

Heath, C. and D. *Switch: How to change things when change is hard.* New York: Broadway Books, 2010.

Wansink, B. *Mindless Eating.* New York: Bantam Dell, 2006.

7. Food is Medicine

Craig, W.J. "Health-promoting properties of common herbs." *American Journal of Clinical Nutrition* 1999 Sept;70(3):491s–9s.

Tapsell, L.C. et al. "Health benefits of herbs and spices: the past, the present, the future." *Medical Journal of Australia* 2006 Aug 21;185(4 Suppl): S4-24.

8. Eat Your Water

Armstrong, L.E. et al. "Mild dehydration affects mood in healthy young women." *Journal of Nutrition* 2012 Feb;142(2):382-8. doi: 10.3945/jn.111.142000

Dennis, E.A. et al. "Water Consumption Increases Weight Loss During a Hypocaloric Diet Intervention in Middle-aged and Older adults." *Obesity* 2010 Feb;18(2):300-7. doi: 10.1038/oby.2009.235

Ingraham, P. "Water Fever and the Fear of Chronic Dehydration: Do we really need eight glasses of water per day?" Feb 20, 2015, https://www.painscience.com/articles/water.php

Saker, P. et al. "Regional brain responses associated with drinking water during thirst and after its satiation." *Proceedings of the National Academy of Sciences of the United States of America* 2014 Apr 8;111(14):5379-84. doi: 10.1073

Smith, M.F. et al. "Effect of Acute Mild Dehydration on Cognitive-Motor Performance in Golf." *Journal of Strength & Conditioning Research* 2012 Nov;26(11):3075-80. doi: 10.1519/JSC.0b013e318245bea7

Valtin, H. "'Drink at least eight glasses of water a day.' Really? Is there scientific evidence for '8 × 8'?" *American Journal of Physiology – Regulatory, Integrative and Comparative Physiology* 2002 Nov;283(5): R993-1004.

9. Take the Eating-In Challenge

Todd, J.E. et al. "The Impact of Food Away From Home on Adult Diet Quality." U.S. Department of Agriculture, Economic

Research Service, February 2010, http://uhs.berkeley.edu/Facstaff/
pdf/healthmatters/FoodAwayFromHome.pdf

10. Eat Yourself Straight

Bowman, K. *Alignment Matters*. Carlsborg, WA: Propriometrics Press,
2013.

11. Good Fat, Bad Fat

"FDA Guidance for Industry: A Food Labeling Guide." http://www.
fda.gov/Food/GuidanceRegulation/GuidanceDocumentsRegulatory-
Information/LabelingNutrition/ucm064911.htm

Mozaffarian, D. et al. "Dietary intake of trans fatty acids and systemic
inflammation in women." *American Journal of Clinical Nutrition* 2004
Apr;79(4):606-12.

Russo, G.L. "Dietary n-6 and n-3 polyunsaturated fatty acids: from
biochemistry to clinical implications in cardiovascular prevention."
Biochemical Pharmacology 2009 Mar 15;77(6):937-46. doi: 10.1016

Siri-Tarino, P.W. et al. "Meta-analysis of prospective cohort studies
evaluating the association of saturated fat with cardiovascular disease."
American Journal of Clinical Nutrition 2010 Mar; 91(3):535-46. doi:
10.3945

12. Don't Have a Cow, Man!

Crovetti, R. et al. "The influence of thermic effect of food on satiety."
European Journal of Clinical Nutrition 1998 Jul;52(7):482-8.

Heaney, R.P. and Layman, D.K. "Amount and type of protein

influences bone health." *American Journal of Clinical Nutrition* 2008. May;87(5):1567S-1570S

13. Drink Coffee. Not Too Much. Mostly Black.

Bhoo-Pathy, N. et al. "Coffee and tea consumption and risk of pre- and postmenopausal breast cancer in the European Prospective Investigation into Cancer and Nutrition (EPIC) cohort study." *Breast Cancer Research* 2015 Jan 31;17:15. doi: 10.1186

Jee, S.H. et al. "Coffee consumption and serum lipids: a meta-analysis of randomized controlled clinical trials." *American Journal of Epidemiology* 2001 Feb 15;153(4):353-62.

Killer, S.C. et al. "No Evidence of Dehydration with Moderate Daily Coffee Intake a counterbalanced cross-over study in a free-living population." *PLOS One* 2014 Jan 9;9(1):e84154. doi: 10.1371

Rego Costa, A.C. et al. "Influence of the dietary intake of medium chain triglycerides on body composition, energy expenditure and satiety: a systematic review." *Nutrición Hospitalaria* 2012 Jan-Feb;27(1):103-8. doi: 10.1590

Ross, G.W. et al. "Association of coffee and caffeine intake with the risk of Parkinson disease." *Journal of the American Medical Association* 2000 May 24-31;283(20):2674-9.

van Dusseldorp, M. et al. "Cholesterol-raising factor from boiled coffee does not pass a paper filter." *Arteriosclerosis, Thrombosis, and Vascular Biology* 1991 May-Jun;11(3):586-93.

Vojdani, A. and Tarash, I. "Cross-Reaction between Gliadin and Different Food and Tissue Antigens." *Food and Nutrition Sciences* 2013; 4: 20-32.

14. Something Fishy This Way Comes

Kaneko, J.J. and Ralston, N.V. "Selenium and mercury in pelagic fish in the central north pacific near Hawaii." *Biological Trace Element Research* 2007 Dec;119(3):242-54.

Kresser, C. "5 Reasons why concerns about mercury in fish are misguided," http://chriskresser.com/5-reasons-why-concerns-about-mercury-in-fish-are-misguided

Kresser, C. "Fukushima Radiation: Is It Still Safe To Eat Fish?" http://chriskresser.com/fukushima-seafood

Lederman, S.A. et al. "Relation between Cord Blood Mercury Levels and Early Child Development in a World Trade Center Cohort," *Environmental Health Perspectives* 2008 Aug;116(8):1085-91. doi: 10.1289

Monterey Bay Aquarium Seafood Watch. http://www.seafoodwatch.org/

Mozaffarian, D. and Rimm, E.B. "Fish Intake, Contaminants, and Human Health – Evaluating the Risks and the Benefits." *Journal of the American Medical Association* 2006 Oct 18;296(15):1885-99.

Nicholas, S. et al. "Evaluation of radiation doses and associated risk from the Fukushima nuclear accident to marine biota and human consumers of seafood." *Proceedings of the National Academy of Sciences* 2013; 110(26): 10670-10675. doi:10.1073

"The Ten Riskiest Foods Regulated by the U.S. Food and Drug Administration," http://www.cspinet.org/new/pdf/cspi_top_10_fda.pdf

Wu, S. et al. "Omega-3 fatty acids intake and risks of dementia and Alzheimer's disease: a meta-analysis." *Neuroscience & Biobehavioral Reviews* 2015 Jan;48:1-9. doi: 10.1016s

16. Odds and Ends and the Anti-Cancer Soup

Brind, J. et al. "Dietary glycine supplementation mimics lifespan extension by dietary methionine restriction in Fisher 344 rats." *FASEB Journal* 2011;25(528.522).

Fallon, S. and Enig, M. *Nourishing Traditions.* Washington, DC: New Trends Publishing, 1999.

Pan, A. et al. "Red Meat Consumption and Mortality: Results from Two Prospective Cohort Studies." *Archives of Internal Medicine* 2012;172(7):555-563. doi:10.1001/archinternmed.2011.2287

17. Ferment Your Food

Ciciarelli, J. *Fermented: A Four Season Approach to Paleo Probiotic Foods.* Las Vegas: Victory Belt, 2013.

Fallon, S. and Enig, M. *Nourishing Traditions.* Washington, DC: New Trends Publishing, 1999.

19. Raw, Cooked, Juiced

Block, G. et al. "Fruit, vegetables, and cancer prevention: a review of the epidemiological evidence." *Nutrition and Cancer* 1992;18(1):1-29.

Carter, P. et al. "Fruit and vegetable intake and incidence of type 2 diabetes mellitus: systematic review and meta-analysis." *BMJ* 2010 Aug 18;341:c4229. doi: 10.1136/bmj.c4229

Dauchet, L. et al. "Fruit and vegetable consumption and risk of stroke: a meta-analysis of cohort studies." *Neurology* 2005 Oct 25;65(8):1193-7.

"Green veg: a one-stop-shop for a healthier life?" https://www.bhf.org.uk/news-from-the-bhf/news-archive/2014/december/dietary-nitrates

Hu, D. et al. "Fruit and vegetable consumption and risk of stroke – a meta-analysis of cohort studies." *Stroke* 2014 Jun;45(6):1613-9. doi: 10.1161/STROKEAHA.114.004836

Lock, K. et al. "The global burden of disease attributable to low consumption of fruit and vegetables: implications for the global strategy on diet." *Bulletin of the World Health Organization* 2005 Feb;83(2):100-8.

Nurmatov, U. et al. "Nutrients and foods for the primary prevention of asthma and allergy: Systematic review and meta-analysis." *Journal of Allergy and Clinical Immunology* 2011 Mar;127(3):724-33.e1-30. doi: 10.1016/j.jaci.2010.11.001

Pavia, M. et al. "Association between fruit and vegetable consumption and oral cancer: a meta-analysis of observational studies." *American Journal of Clinical Nutrition* 2006 May;83(5):1126-34.

Pomerleau, J. et al. "The burden of cardiovascular disease and cancer attributable to low fruit and vegetable intake in the European Union: differences between old and new Member States." *Public Health Nutrition* 2006 Aug;9(5):575-83.

Robinson, J. *Eating on the Wild Side – The Missing Link to Optimum Health*. New York: Little, Brown, 2013.

van't Veer, P. et al. "Fruits and vegetables in the prevention of cancer and cardiovascular disease." *Public Health Nutrition* 2000 Mar;3(1):103-7.

20. Just Look, You Don't Have to Touch

Richman, J. and Sheth, A. *What's Your Poo Telling You?* San Francisco: Chronicle Books, 2007.

Sangu, P.K. et al. "A study on Tailabindu pariksha – An ancient Ayurvedic method of urine examination as a diagnostic and prognostic tool." *Ayu* 2011 Jan;32(1):76-81. doi: 10.4103/0974-8520.85735

"Urine Color Chart," http://health.clevelandclinic.org/2013/10/what-the-color-of-your-urine-says-about-you-infographic/

"What Exactly Are Normal Stools?," https://www.gutsense.org/constipation/normal_stools.html

21. Walking Like Nature Intended

Dimeo, F. et al. "Benefits from aerobic exercise in patients with major depression: a pilot study." 2001 Apr;35(2):114-7.

Krall, E.A. and Dawson-Hughes, B. "Walking is related to bone density and rates of bone loss." *American Journal of Medicine* 1994 Jan;96(1):20-6.

Oppezzo, M. and Schwartz, D.L. "Give your ideas some legs: the positive effect of walking on creative thinking." *Journal of Experimental Psychology: Learning, Memory, and Cognition* 2014 Jul;40(4):1142-52. doi: 10.1037/a0036577

Williams, P.T. and Thompson, P.D. "Walking versus running for hypertension, cholesterol, and diabetes mellitus risk reduction." *Arteriosclerosis, Thrombosis, and Vascular Biology* 2013 May;33(5):1085-91. doi: 10.1161/ATVBAHA.112.300878

22. Meet Your Feet

Bergmann, G. et al. "Influence of shoes and heel strike on the loading of the hip joint." *Journal of Biomechanics* 1995 Jul;28(7):817-27.

Bowman, K. *Whole Body Barefoot.* Carlsborg, WA: Propriometrics Press, 2015.

Bowman, K. *Every Woman's Guide to Foot Pain Relief.* Dallas: BenBella Books, 2011.

Goss, D.L. and Gross, M.T. "Relationships among self-reported shoe type, footstrike pattern, and injury incidence." *Army Medical Department Journal* 2012 Oct-Dec:25-30.

McClanahan, R. "How Healthy Are Your Feet?" Natural Running Center. August 2013, https://cdn.nwfootankle.com/editor/files/208/NRCBooklet-HealthyFeet-rc3.pdf

Robbins, S.E. and Gouw, G.J. "Athletic footwear: unsafe due to perceptual illusions." *Medicine & Science in Sports & Exercise* 1991 Feb;23(2):217-24.

Rossi, W.A. "Footwear: The Primary Cause of Foot Disorders." *Podiatry Management* 2001 Feb:129–38.

Rossi, W.A. "Why Shoes Make 'Normal' Gait Impossible." *Podiatry Management* 1999 Mar:50–61.

24. Goodbye, Turkey Head

Enwemeka, C.S. et al. "Postural Correction in Persons with Neck Pain. II. Integrated Electromyography of the Upper Trapezius in Three Simulated Neck Positions." *Journal of Orthopaedic & Sports Physical Therapy* 1986;8(5):240-2.

Griegel-Morris, P. et al. "Incidence of common postural abnormalities in the cervical, shoulder, and thoracic regions and their association with pain in two age groups of healthy subjects." *Physical Therapy Journal* 1992 Jun;72(6):425-31.

Silva, A.G. et al. "Head Posture and Neck Pain of Chronic Nontraumatic Origin: A Comparison Between Patients and Pain-Free Persons." *Archives of Physical Medicine and Rehabilitation* 2009 Apr;90(4):669-74. doi: 10.1016/j.apmr.2008.10.018

25. Finding Your Fitness Path

Batra, P. et al. "Eating behaviors as predictors of weight loss in a 6-month weight loss intervention." *Obesity* 2013 Nov;21(11):2256-63. doi: 10.1002/oby.20404

DiPietro, L. et al. "Three 15-min bouts of moderate postmeal walking significantly improves 24-h glycemic control in older people at risk for impaired glucose tolerance." *Diabetes Care* 2013 Oct;36(10):3262-8. doi: 10.2337/dc13-0084

Flegal, K.M. et al. "Association of all-cause mortality with overweight and obesity using standard body mass index categories: a systematic review and meta-analysis." *Journal of the American Medical Association* 2013 Jan 2;309(1):71-82. doi: 10.1001/jama.2012.113905

Lang, J.J. et al. "Sit less, stand more: A randomized point-of-decision prompt intervention to reduce sedentary time." *Preventive Medicine* 2015 Apr;73:67-9. doi: 10.1016/j.ypmed.2015.01.026

O'Keefe, J.H. et al. "Potential Adverse Cardiovascular Effects From Excessive Endurance Exercise." *Mayo Clinic Proceedings* 2012 Jun; 87(6): 587–595. doi:10.1016/j.mayocp.2012.04.005

Williams, P.T. and Thompson, P.D. "Walking versus running for hypertension, cholesterol, and diabetes mellitus risk reduction." *Arteriosclerosis, Thrombosis, and Vascular Biology* 2013 May;33(5):1085-91. doi: 10.1161/ATVBAHA.112.300878

27. Move Like a Baby

Anderson, T. *Original Strength*. Maitland, FL: Xulon Press, 2013.

Frank, C. et al. "Dynamic neuromuscular stabilization & sports rehabilitation," *International Journal of Sports Physical Therapy* 2013 Feb;8(1):62-73

Kolar, P. et al. "Postural function of the diaphragm in persons with and without chronic low back pain," *Journal of Orthopaedic & Sports Physical Therapy* 2012 Apr;42(4):352-62. doi: 10.2519/jospt.2012.3830

Kuo, Y.L. et al. "The influence of wakeful prone positioning on motor development during the early life," *Journal of Developmental & Behavioral Pediatrics* 2008 Oct;29(5):367-76. doi: 10.1097/DBP.0b013e3181856d54

Myers, T. "KQ = Kinesthetic Quotient = Physical Intelligence," 2005, http://bti.edu/pdfs/Myers_Kinesthetic-Quotient.pdf

29. Bulletproof Your Low Back

Bowman, K. *Alignment Matters*. Carlsborg, WA: Propriometrics Press, 2013.

Bowman, K. *Move Your DNA*. Carlsborg, WA: Propriometrics Press, 2015.

30. Roll With It

Cheatham, S.W. et al. "The effects of self-myofascial release using a foam roll or roller massager on joint range of motion, muscle recovery, and performance: a systematic review." *Journal of Orthopaedic and Sports Physical Therapy* 2015 Nov;10(6):827-38.

Grieve, R. et al. "The immediate effect of bilateral self myofascial release on the plantar surface of the feet on hamstring and lumbar spine flexibility: a pilot randomised controlled trial." *Journal of Bodywork and Movement Therapies* 2015 Jul;19(3):544-52. doi: 10.1016/j.jbmt.2014.12.004

LeMoon, K. "Terminology used in fascia research." *Journal of Bodywork and Movement Therapies* 2008 Jul: 204-212.

31. Squat Your Way to Health

"Ability to sit and rise from the floor as a predictor of all-cause mortality." (video) *European Journal of Cardiovascular Prevention*, http://bit.ly/1v1Qf1K

Brito, L. et al. "Ability to sit and rise from the floor as a predictor of all-cause mortality." *European Journal of Preventive Cardiology* 2014 Jul;21(7):892-8. doi: 10.1177/2047487312471759

Sikirov, D. "Comparison of Straining During Defecation in Three Positions, Results and Implications for Human Health." *Digestive Diseases and Sciences* 2003 Jul;48(7):1201-5.

32. Let It Go

Levine, P. *In an Unspoken Voice.* Berkeley, CA: North Atlantic Books, 2010.

Levine, P. *Waking the Tiger.* Berkeley, CA: North Atlantic Books, 1997.

33. Explore Your Breathing

Bowman, K. *Diastasis Recti.* Carlsborg, WA: Propriometrics Press, 2015.

Chaitow, L., Gilbert, C. and Bradley, D. *Recognizing and Treating Breathing Disorders: A Multidisciplinary Approach.* New York: Churchill Livingstone/Elsevier, 2014.

Kolar, P. et al. "Postural function of the diaphragm in persons with and without chronic low back pain." *Journal of Orthopaedic & Sports Physical Therapy* 2012 Apr;42(4):352-62. doi: 10.2519/jospt.2012.3830

"Nose breathing versus mouth breathing; nose breathing is Optimal. See why and how below," breathing.com/articles/nose-breathing.htm

34. Quiet Time

Abey-Wickrama, I. et al. "Mental hospital admissions and aircraft noise." *Lancet* 1970 Feb 28;1(7644):467-8.

EPA, "Noise Pollution," https://www.epa.gov/clean-air-act-overview/title-iv-noise-pollutionArticles on noise pollution, noiseoff.com, http://www.noiseoff.org/library.php#articles

Hodgetts, W.E. et al. "The Effects of Listening Environment and Earphone Style on Preferred Listening Levels of Normal Hearing Adults Using an MP3 Player." *Ear and Hearing* 2007 Jun;28(3):290-7.

Meecham, W.C. and Smith, H.G. "Effects of jet aircraft noise on mental hospital admissions." *British Journal of Audiology* 1977; 11: 81–5.

Morita, E. et al. "Psychological effects of forest environments on healthy adults: Shinrin-yoku (forest-air bathing, walking) as a possible method of stress reduction." *Public Health* 2007 Jan;121(1):54-63. Epub 2006 Oct 20.

Shinrin-yoku, http://www.shinrin-yoku.org/

35. Stand Up for Yourself

Dunstan, D.W. et al. "Breaking up prolonged sitting reduces postprandial glucose and insulin responses." *Diabetes Care* 35: 976–983, 2012.

Healy, G.N. et al. "Breaks in sedentary time: beneficial associations with metabolic risk." *Diabetes Care* 2008 Apr,31(4):661-6. doi: 10.2337/dc07-2046

Olsen, R.H. et al. "Metabolic responses to reduced daily steps in healthy nonexercising men." *Journal of the American Medical Association* 299: 1261-1263.

Wilmot, E.G. et al. "Sedentary time in adults and the association with diabetes, cardiovascular disease and death: systematic review and meta-analysis." *Diabetologia* 2012 Nov;55(11):2895-905. doi: 10.1007/s00125-012-2677-z

36. Intermittent Fasting

"Fasting and weight loss," http://www.marksdailyapple.com/fasting-weight-loss

Halberg, N. et al. "Effect of intermittent fasting and refeeding on insulin action in healthy men." *Journal of Applied Physiology* (1985). 2005 Dec;99(6):2128-36

Lee, C. and Longo, V.D. "Fasting vs dietary restriction in cellular protection and cancer treatment: from model organisms to patients," *Oncogene* 2011 Jul 28;30(30):3305-16. doi: 10.1038/onc.2011.91

Siegel, I. et al. "Effects of short-term dietary restriction on survival of mammary ascites tumor-bearing rats." *Cancer Investigation* 1988;6(6):677-80.

37. Level Up Your Vacation

Chikani, V. et al. "Vacations improve mental health among rural women: the Wisconsin Rural Women's Health Study." *WMJ* 2005 Aug;104(6):20-3.

Gump, B.B. and Matthews, K.A. "Are vacations good for your health? The 9-year mortality experience after the multiple risk factor intervention trial." *Psychosomatic Medicine* 2000 Sep-Oct;62(5):608-12.

Park, B.J. et al. "The physiological effects of Shinrin-yoku (taking in the forest atmosphere or forest bathing): evidence from field experiments in 24 forests across Japan." *Environmental Health and Preventive Medicine* 2010 Jan;15(1):18-26. doi: 10.1007/s12199-009-0086-9

38. Your Dynamic Office

Dunstan, D.W. et al. "Breaking up prolonged sitting reduces postprandial glucose and insulin responses." *Diabetes Care* 2012 May;35(5):976-83. doi: 10.2337/dc11-1931

Hamilton, M.T. et al. "Role of Low Energy Expenditure and Sitting in Obesity, Metabolic Syndrome, Type 2 Diabetes, and Cardiovascular Disease." *Diabetes* 2007 Nov;56(11):2655-67. Epub 2007 Sep 7

Pomodoro Technique, http://pomodorotechnique.com

39. Furniture Minimalism

Brito, L. et al. "Ability to sit and rise from the floor as a predictor of all-cause mortality." *European Journal of Preventive Cardiology* 2014 Jul;21(7):892-8. doi: 10.1177/2047487312471759

Hewes, G. "World Distribution of Certain Postural Habits." *American Anthropologist*, New Series, 1955 Apr;57(2):231–44. doi: 10.1525/aa.1955.57.2.02a00040

40. Are You Sleep-Deprived?

NIH, "Cyrcadian Rhythms Facts Sheet," https://www.nigms.nih.gov/Education/Pages/Factsheet_CircadianRhythms.aspx

Sapolsky, R. *Why Zebras Don't Get Ulcers.* New York: Henry Holt Books, 1994.

Wiley, T.S. *Lights Out: Sleep, Sugar, and Survival.* New York: Pocket Books, 2000.

41. Sharpen Your Vision

He, M. et al. "Effect of Time Spent Outdoors at School on the Development of Myopia Among Children in China, A Randomized Clinical Trial." *JAMA* 2015;314(11):1142-1148. doi:10.1001/jama.2015.10803

Huang, H.M. et al. "The Association between Near Work Activities and Myopia in Children – A Systematic Review and Meta-Analysis." *PLOS One* 2015 Oct 20;10(10):e0140419. doi: 10.1371/journal.pone.0140419

Jacques, P.F. et al. "Long-term nutrient intake and 5-year change in nuclear lens opacities." *JAMA Ophthalmology* 2005 Apr;123(4):517-2

Mitchell, P. et al. "Nutritional factors in the development of age-related eye disease." *Asia Pacific Journal of Clinical Nutrition* 2003 12 (Suppl): S5.

Simons, H.D. and Gassler, P.A. "Vision anomalies and reading skill: a meta-analysis of the literature," *American Journal of Optometry and Physiological Optics* 1988 Nov;65(11):893-904

Tan, J.S. et al. "Dietary Antioxidants and the Long-Term Incidence of Age-Related Macular Degeneration: The Blue Mountains Eye Study." *Ophthalmology* 2008 Feb;115(2):334-41.

43. Read the Small Print

EWG, "A benchmark investigation of industrial chemicals,

pollutants and pesticides in umbilical cord blood," http://www.ewg.org/research/body-burden-pollution-newborns

Wolfe, L. "Skintervention," http://skinterventionguide.org

44. Meditate on This

Chiesa, A. and Serretti, A. "Mindfulness-based stress reduction for stress management in healthy people: a review and meta-analysis." *Journal of Alternative and Complementary Medicine* 2009 May;15(5):593-600. doi: 10.1089/acm.2008.0495

Goyal, M. et al. "Meditation programs for psychological stress and well-being: a systematic review and meta-analysis." *JAMA Internal Medicine* 2014;174(3):357-368. doi:10.1001/jamainternmed.2013.13018

Grossman, P. et al. "Mindfulness-based stress reduction and health benefits. A meta-analysis." *Journal of Psychosomatic Research* 2004 Jul;57(1):35-43

Payne, P. et al. "Somatic experiencing: using interoception and proprioception as core elements of trauma therapy," *Frontiers in Psychology* 2015; 6: 93, doi: 10.3389/fpsyg.2015.00093

45. Walk More Today

Williams, P.T. and Thompson, P.D. "Walking Versus Running for Hypertension, Cholesterol, and Diabetes Mellitus Risk Reduction." *Journal of Arteriosclerosis, Thrombosis, and Vascular Biology* 2013 May;33(5):1085-91. doi: 10.1161/ATVBAHA.112.300878

46. Confessions of a Massage Addict

Craniosacral Therapy, http://www.upledger.com

Jacobs, G.D. et al. "The effects of short term flotation REST on relaxation: a controlled study." *Health Psychology* 1984;3(2):99-112.

Massage Therapy Glossary, http://www.massagetherapy.com/glossary

47. Yoga is Not Just for Yogis

Kelder, P. *The Five Tibetan Rites of Rejuvenation*. New York: Doubleday, 2007.

50. The E-Detox

Kansas State University, "Mental break: Work-life balance needed for recovery from job stress." https://www.k-state.edu/media/news-releases/feb13/worklifebal20513.html

ICMPA and students at the Phillip Merrill College of Journalism, University of Maryland, College Park, "A Day Without Media," https://withoutmedia.wordpress.com

Misra, S. et al. "The iPhone Effect, The Quality of In-Person Social Interactions in the Presence of Mobile Devices." *Environment and Behavior* (Impact Factor: 1.27). 2014 Jul; 48(2). DOI: 10.1177/0013916514539755

Ophira, E. et al. "Cognitive control in media multitaskers." *Proceedings of the National Academy of Sciences*, 2009 Aug 25;106(33).

Screen Free Week, http://www.screenfree.org

Tecmark. "Tecmark survey finds average user picks up their smartphone 221 times a day." http://www.tecmark.co.uk/smartphone-usage-data-uk-2014

51. I Have Needs

Perel, E. *Mating in Captivity.* New York: HarperCollins, 2007.

52. Get Dirty

Chalquist, C. "A look at the ecotherapy research evidence." June 2009, Ecophycology, http://sustainability.emory.edu/uploads/articles/2009/08/2009080315530099/ecotheraphyeco.2009.0003.lowlink.pdf_v03.pdf

INDEX

Bowman, Katy 179-180, 224

breathing 56, 72-74, 146, 160, 183, 200, 209-211, 217-218, 226, 230, 241, 251, 253, 254, 258, 260-266, 300, 317, 343, 348, 352-353, 356, 361-365, 377

broth xiii, xiv, 9, 10, 28, 32, 35, 56, 67, 118, 120-123

bunion 164-167, 175-176

butter 12, 48, 77-85, 98

C

caffeine 62, 97-101

cancer 28, 56-58, 95, 104, 113, 117, 134, 275, 306, 310, 331

carbs/carbohydrates 11, 40, 68, 86, 89, 91, 93, 102, 130, 135, 290, 320

"cardio" (style of exercise) 188-191, 195, 294, 347

cardiovascular system/health, 52-53, 73, 134, 154, 156-157, 165, 188-191, 195, 269, 294-295, 307, 310, 347

carnitas 7-13, 27, 131

chicken 7-11, 19, 22, 25, 33, 36, 46, 55, 56, 68, 86, 90-93, 104, 108, 114, 120-123, 129-131, 192

children 14, 22-23, 39, 49, 60, 105, 120, 136, 172, 179, 186, 187, 192, 197-200, 216, 241-242, 250, 273, 286, 289-291, 301, 313, 318-324, 333, 349, 376-377, 386, 388

Chinese medicine, *see* medicine, traditional/holistic

cholesterol 55, 88, 96, 98, 136, 347

circadian rhythm 309-313

coconut milk 35, 46, 55, 100-101, 114, 131

coconut oil 12, 46-48, 81-82, 98, 330, 334-335

coconut sugar 113

coffee 62, 97-101

I

immune system/immunity, 34, 40, 42, 51, 56-58, 79, 88, 124, 136,
143, 264, 306, 327

intimacy 378, 390-394

J

journal/journaling 1-4, 14, 43, 49, 69, 84, 94, 116, 122, 206, 314,
336, 350, 369, 371, 373, 380, 394, 398, 402

K

kids, *see* children

kimchi 126, 140, 240

kombucha 46, 126-127

L

labels (on packaging) 17-21, 25, 80-81, 84, 113, 125, 126, 333, 336

Loomis, Barbara 26, 144

Lopes, Kaisa, PhD 52-54, 58

losing weight, *see* weight management

M

massage 26, 146, 170-171, 175, 224-225, 230-238, 291-292, 334,
346, 351-357, 376

medicine, chemical/allopathic 149, 150, 156, 224-225, 251, 265, 278,
333, 344, 347, 354, 375-376

medicine, traditional/holistic xi, 50-59, 62, 146-147, 151, 224-225,
352-357, 375-376

meditation 2, 340-344, 369, 371, 376, 380

mercury 102-105, 108

U

urinary system 58

urine *see* pee

V

vacation 2, 284-293, 317, 321, 349, 388

vitamins (found in food) 20, 68, 113, 136, 143, 187, 317, 319, 320

vitamins (pill) 19

W

Walker, Matt 310

walking xi, 3, 34, 50, 87, 136, 154-163, 165, 167-171, 172-173, 176-177, 180, 182, 186-195, 199-200, 207-209, 216-222, 223-225, 241, 255, 264, 273-277, 291, 296-298, 301, 303, 317, 322-323, 326, 342-343, 345-350, 352-353, 367-371, 377, 380, 385, 395

water (in your diet) 38-43, 55, 60-65, 97, 151, 243, 274, 367, 377, 382

weight management xi, 17, 27, 29, 40, 44-45, 62—63, 66-69, 72, 87-94, 98, 102, 113, 129, 188-195, 264, 273, 274-276, 278, 283, 284, 295, 307, 345, 347, 359, 360, 374-375, 386

Wolfe, Liz 336

Y

yoga 192, 230

Yoga Tune Up© 233, 237, 260, 273, 290-291, 303, 326, 353, 355, 358-366, 370

yogurt 26, 46, 48, 53-57, 90-93, 110, 114, 124-127

ACKNOWLEDGMENTS

Creating this book would have been impossible without the generous support of our teachers, and the rich collaboration with our students. For each lesson we wrote for you and with you, we also learned ourselves. We learned from every interview, every study that we read, and from each conversation with one of our experts. Most of all, we learned from our Eat Well, Move Well tribe – our readers, students, clients, family, and friends. Thank you.

This book contains the wisdom of so many, and is built on encouragement from even more.

Doctor Spencer Nadolsky, Katy Bowman, Dan Pardi, Dr. Stephan Guyenet, Dr. Mike T. Nelson, Elmira Nam, Shannon Leith, Barbara Loomis, Chef Nikolay Dimitrov, Dr. Kaisa Lopes, Liz Wolfe, Jo Robinson, Alexandra Denzel, the guys from Freakonomics Radio, Dr. Karl Nadolsky, Jill Miller, Paul Daniels, Mark Sisson, Alan Aragon, Jake Steiner, Dan John, Jamie Oliver, and Galina's father, Ivan Ivanov.

And for the ongoing help and encouragement, Lou Schuler, Dave Sisler, Scott Schaffer, Dave Tropeano, Debbie Beane, Ken Scott, Michael Curran, Dale Equitz, Lisa Steinberger, Breena Maggio, Carl Sinclair, Lisa Gillispie, Lois Laynee, Abi Blakeslee, Michael Rintala, Sean Hendrickson, Kevin Tumlinson, Jo and Ashley Handal, Jodee Nelson, Angelo Coppola, Mark Fisher, Greg and Lani Rager, Nick Bromberg, Krista Scott-Dixon, Dani Hemmat, Skyler Richter, Paul Constantine, Jim Governale, Bill Hartman, Emre Harputlu-oglu, Jeanne Cameron, Autumn Lewis, and coffee.

ABOUT THE AUTHORS

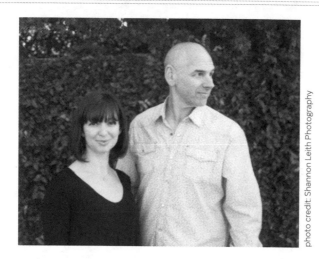

photo credit: Shannon Leith Photography

International wellness coaches Galina and Roland Denzel help people achieve their health goals through simple solutions brought about by easily manageable changes. They share a practice in Southern California, and reach thousands more via their website, eatwellmovewell.com. Between them they've published numerous books, including *Man on Top*, their weight loss guide based on Roland's own 75-pound weight loss journey, *The Real Food Reset*, a practical 30-day guide to reconnecting with real food, and several whole-food cookbooks. Along with their training in corrective exercise, nutrition, and coaching, they bring a wealth of personal experience, warmth, humor, and a healthy dose of wisdom to the table.

Roland and Galina constantly post examples of an Eat Well, Move Well, Live Well life on their social media channels. Follow them to see the many tips in this book in action!

Facebook.com/EatWellMoveWellOnline

Twitter @rolanddenzel

Instagram @galinadenzel